OPTOMETRIC MANAGEMENT
OF VISUAL HANDICAP

Modern Optometry

SERIES EDITOR

R. FLETCHER

MScTech, FBCO, FBOA, HD, FSMC (Hons), DOrth, DCLP, FAAO

Emeritus Professor, City University, London

Docent II, Kongsberg Inginør Høgskole, Kongsberg, Norge

Optometric Management
of Visual Handicap

HELEN FARRALL

PhD, MSc, FBCO

Principal Optometrist, Coventry and Warwickshire Hospital
Coventry

Blackwell
Science

© 1991 by Helen Farrall

Blackwell Science Ltd
Editorial Offices:
Osney Mead, Oxford OX2 0EL
25 John Street, London WC1N 2BL
23 Ainslie Place, Edinburgh EH3 6AJ
350 Main Street, Malden
  MA 02148 5018, USA
54 University Street, Carlton
  Victoria 3053, Australia
10, rue Casimir Delavigne
  75006 Paris, France

Other Editorial Offices:

Blackwell Wissenschafts-Verlag GmbH
Kurfürstendamm 57
10707 Berlin, Germany

Blackwell Science KK
MG Kodenmacho Building
7–10 Kodenmacho Nihombashi
Chuo-ku, Tokyo 104, Japan

First published 1991
Reprinted 1996, 1998

Set by Setrite Typesetters Ltd, Hong Kong
Printed and bound in Great Britain by
the University Press, Cambridge

The Blackwell Science logo is a
trade mark of Blackwell Science Ltd,
registered at the United Kingdom
Trade Marks Registry

DISTRIBUTORS

Marston Book Services Ltd
PO Box 269
Abingdon
Oxon OX14 4YN
(*Orders:* Tel: 01235 465500
        Fax: 01235 465555)

USA
Blackwell Science, Inc.
Commerce Place
350 Main Street
Malden, MA 02148 5018
(*Orders:* Tel: 800 759 6102
                781 388 8250
        Fax: 781 388 8255)

Canada
Login Brothers Book Company
324 Saulteaux Crescent
Winnipeg, Manitoba R3J 3T2
(*Orders:* Tel: 204 224-4068)

Australia
Blackwell Science Pty Ltd
54 University Street
Carlton, Victoria 3053
(*Orders:* Tel: 03 9347 0300
        Fax: 03 9347 5001)

A catalogue record for this title
is available from the British Library

ISBN 0-632-02774-6

Contents

Preface

Visual defects are predominantly caused by genetic factors or age-related disease processes. Thus, despite major advances in the medical and surgical management of ocular and systemic disease, increased longevity is inevitably resulting in greater numbers of visually impaired people within the population.

At the same time, the visual complexity and demands of everyday life are increasing, and attitudes and expectations concerning blindness and partial sight are changing. Despite impaired vision, children are encouraged to tackle a full school curriculum, adults to seek employment, and the elderly to maintain an independent lifestyle.

Greater expectations among greater numbers of visually impaired people present an ever increasing challenge to the various care and support professions involved.

The scope of so-called 'low vision aid' work has enlarged considerably in recent years. This book is a result of time spent in general optometric practice, plus many years' clinical work in the Hospital Eye Service, liaison with teachers and social services, and experience of training and examining pre-registration level optometry students.

The aim is to fill a perceived need to place the students' theoretical knowledge into a broader clinical context and provide the technical information and ideas to encourage the experienced optometrist to expand the service offered to visually impaired patients. The optical and assessment information will also be of value to specialist teachers, social workers and other associated professionals, who should ideally have an appreciation of the range and limitations of optical low vision aids.

The book takes a wide clinical view of the subject. The intention is to integrate the relatively specialised optometric assessment and provision of optical aids and spectacles with a broader, advisory approach. The role of non-optical aids, lighting and colour is emphasised, in conjunction with the need to appreciate the various educational, work or social circumstances involved in the overall management of an individual person's visual handicap.

Several appendices provide valuable data to support the information and discussion found in the text. References, of a clinical, rather than excessively theoretical nature, have been limited to those which should be most helpful as well as reasonably available.

The photographs are predominantly the work of Martin Hewitt, of the Medical Illustration Department, Coventry and Warwickshire Hospital. My sincere thanks for his patience as well as for his considerable professional expertise.

I am indebted to manufacturers for permission to reproduce the technical specification of product ranges. Also to Richard Bignall, Headmaster, his staff and pupils at Exhall Grange School, and to my colleagues and patients at Coventry and Warwickshire Hospital. My thanks also to Professor Robert Fletcher for much helpful guidance during the preparation of the text; to Ann Fearn for secretarial assistance; to Richard Miles and the whole production team at Blackwell Science.

The greatest debt of gratitude however, is due to David, for willingly taking over as chef and chief domestic organiser, without whose support the book would never have been possible.

Helen Farrall
1991

CHAPTER 1

Blindness and Partial Sight: An Overview

1.1   Introduction

Blindness and visual impairment in the technically developed countries is largely an age-related problem. The blindness rate within the population as a whole is of the order of 200 per 100 000. However, 70% of those registered blind in Britain are over 70 years of age. Increasing longevity and improved medical control of such diseases as diabetes and hypertension are inevitably producing a steady increase in the demand for assistance, information and services for the visually impaired.

In the technically developing countries the major factors contributing to blindness are infection and malnutrition, conditions which are both treatable and preventable. In such countries the ratio of non-infectious:infectious causes of blindness is 1:35, compared to 11:1 in the 'developed' world (Tarizzo, 1972).

Developing countries' prime need is for water purification programmes, improved hygiene and better medical facilities. Optical and rehabilitation services for the visually impaired, while clearly desirable, will understandably be afforded low priority. Statistical information gathering procedures are also minimal, such that in many countries there is no real way of assessing the scale of the problem or even the numbers of blind and severely visually handicapped individuals in the population.

A 1966 study by the World Health Organization found no less than 65 different definitions of the level of visual function at which a person could be legally registered as blind. The situation is further complicated by the fact that some countries recognise the concept of 'low vision' or 'partial sight' as a separate entity from that of legal blindness. Other countries recognise only two groups − the seeing and the legally blind. The legally blind group itself is far from homogeneous. It contains people with widely differing degrees and types of visual loss. Sorsby (1966) surveying blind registration in England and Wales found only 3.4% with no perception of light. The overwhelming majority of legally blind people have some degree of residual vision.

The intention of this book is to provide information and advice appropriate both to students and qualified optometrists, and to others professionally involved in work with visually impaired people. While there are inevitably some technical sections concerning lens systems and design, the text stresses the need for a broadly-based 'management' approach to the problems posed by defective sight.

The text covers the clinical examination and assessment appropriate for adults and children with impaired vision, before considering the availability and evaluation of optical aids. The importance of lighting is emphasised, as are many other non-optical methods of assisting a person make optimum use of residual vision and minimise the handicapping effects of poor sight. Blind and partial sight registration criteria and procedures and post-registration statutory provisions are also reviewed.

The information is designed to be of relevance whether dealing with mild visual problems or assisting people with very limited residual sight.

1.2   Impairment – disability – handicap

All registered blind and partially-sighted people have some disorder and impairment of their eyes and/or visual pathways, i.e. they suffer from some congenital or acquired disorder which interferes with the normal function of the structure.

This visual impairment produces disability, i.e. a loss or reduction of the individual's ability to perform certain tasks.

Disability commonly gives rise to some degree of handicap. It should be appreciated that impairment, disability and handicap are not synonymous. 'Disorder' or 'impairment' are appropriate within a medical framework. In measuring visual acuity, visual field, colour vision, etc., and comparing with a previously agreed normal level, one is specifying the degree of visual impairment.

On the other hand, one has only to have a very slight acquaintance with visually impaired people to realise that individuals with very similar visual acuity and field measurements respond to their disorders in widely differing ways.

Disability and handicap on the other hand are social, not medical concepts. They must be viewed in the context of the circumstances of the individual's lifestyle. For some, an inability to read small print is a massive disability. To others it is only a minor irritant. Similarly, reduction of distance vision below driving standard may be a crippling handicap to one person and inconsequential to another.

Handicap implies that the person is at a disadvantage with respect to his own expectations or those of the society within which he lives. The degree of handicap thus relates to the level of expectation. It is a complex interrelationship between the person and his surroundings, involving his own experiences, motivation and intelligence, with those of his family, school, employer and so on.

For example, individuals with a congenital ocular problem and those with an acquired defect, who previously had normal sight, often respond quite differently to optical aids. The first group will generally view the aid, limitations notwithstanding, as an advance on their normal unaided situation. Their attitude may well be critical and demanding but it is fundamentally a positive response.

The second group, while appreciating that the aid does improve the clarity of an object is understandably inclined to make comparison, not with their present visually impaired state, but with the situation 'as it used to be' before their vision deteriorated.

Someone who has never been able to read a newspaper may be very satisfied with a magnifier which enables him to do so, even though only a few words are visible at a time and the reading speed is naturally rather slow. If, however, the person with an acquired defect was in the habit of devouring acres of newsprint on a Sunday morning, that same magnifying aid might well be rejected. Although technically enabling the person to see the print, the limited field of view may well be felt to be so overwhelmingly inferior to the previous experience of normal reading that it renders the aid unacceptable.

This type of person will be much more acutely aware of the visual disability and feel much more handicapped by it. All you can offer or suggest is naturally inferior to the normal vision lost. It can be difficult to deal with this understandable, but counterproductive, negative attitude. Considerable amounts of patient determination and encouragement on the practitioner's part may be required if the negative response is to be overcome.

The problem is exacerbated in cases of rapid onset visual loss. A person suffering sudden severe reduction or loss of vision generally experiences feelings of anger, followed by anxiety and depression. This requires substantial support and councelling from medical, welfare, rehabilitation and employment services. Sadly, despite its statutory framework, provision of services for the blind and partially sighted is patchy and often woefully inadequate.

1.3   Registration criteria in Britain

1.3.1   The BD8/BP1 form

Decisions regarding blindness and partial sight registration are made by a consultant ophthalmologist who completes form BD8 in England and Wales and form BP1 in Scotland. The fee for completing the registration document is paid by the relevant local health authority.

Full details of the registration documents and the legal criteria defining blindness and partial sight may be found in Appendix 1.

1.3.2   Definition of blindness

The National Assistance Act 1948, defines a blind person as being someone *'so blind as to be unable to perform any work for which eyesight is essential'*. In considering this definition there are two important points to be noted:

(1) The test is not whether the person is unable to pursue his ordinary occupation or any particular occupation, but whether he is too blind to perform any work for which eyesight is essential; and
(2) Only visual conditions are to be taken into account. Other physical or mental conditions are to be disregarded.

The corrected visual acuity levels given for guidance are:

Group 1 — below 3/60 Snellen or below 1/18 Snellen if testing at the closer distance, with a full field.
Group 2 — 3/60, but below 6/60 with a significantly contracted field.
Group 3 — 6/60 Snellen or better, with a gross visual field contraction, particularly in the lower field.

1.3.3 Definition of partial sight

There is no statutory definition of partial sight in the 1948 National Assistance Act. The Department of Health advise that persons may be considered to be partially sighted if *'they are substantially and permanently handicapped by defective vision'*. The defective sight may be of congenital or acquired origin, and brings the person within the scope of the welfare services provided by the local authority. Visually impaired children are now assessed individually by the education departments in terms of their special educational needs.
   Guideline visual acuity levels for partial sight registration are taken as:

(1) 3/60 up to 6/60 with a full field.
(2) up to 6/24 with moderate field contraction, media opacities or aphakia.
(3) 6/18 or better with a gross field defect.

Knowledge of registration criteria and the statutory benefits and entitlements consequent upon registration is necessary if one is to give accurate advice to patients. Students will need the information for examination purposes!
   If handled insensitively blind registration can be a devastating blow to people, leaving them feeling that they have reached 'the end of the road'. On the other hand it can be proposed in a positive way, as a means of access to improved financial, support and mobility services, with the aim of improving the quality of life; not 'writing them off' as being beyond help.

1.4 Post-registration procedures and statutory provisions for assistance

A redesigned BD8 form came into use in England and Wales on 1 April 1990. The new document is in five parts, and like its Scottish counterpart the BP1, now includes a section to be signed by the patient, giving consent to the disclosure of the visual details to the local Social Services Department. This knowledge of the VA (visual acuity), visual field and duration of the visual disability is of great help to the specialist social workers and mobility officers involved. Unfortunately the form makes no reference to the near acuity – a serious omission in the case of children in view of its obvious educational implication.

Details of the patient's actual ocular or systemic medical diagnosis are contained in Part 5 of the form. This information goes only to the patient's GP, not to social services. In an anonymous form (i.e. without the name and address) this section is also sent for statistical purposes to the Office of Population Censuses and Surveys. (Fig. 1.1.)

The patient is also given a copy of the new BD8 to retain. This is a new provision which should prove very beneficial when people move to a new local authority area. At present the information/paperwork tends not to keep up!

Once the person's local Social Service Department has received the completed BD8 form, the information must be passed on to other agencies as appropriate. (Fig. 1.2.)

The National Assistance Act 1948 requires Local Authorities to keep registers of disabled persons resident within their area. Notification of registration will thus need to be given to whoever is responsible for the clerical compilation of the registers. This may be the Social Service Department itself or the office of the District Medical Officer.

Notification of registration should be sent to the Department of Employment in the case of a person of working age seeking employment, with similar

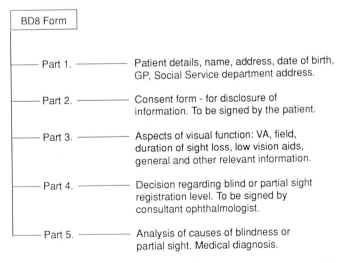

Fig. 1.1 Summary of BD8 form for use in England and Wales, introduced in April 1990.

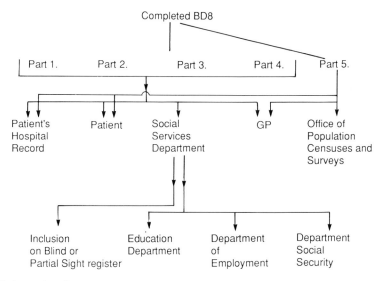

Fig. 1.2 Information flow following completion of BD8 form.

notification to the Department of Social Security (DSS) in the case of persons receiving income support.

Under the terms of the 1981 Education Act the health authority must inform the local education department of any child who is likely to have 'special educational needs'. The child need not actually be registered blind or partially sighted at that stage, but local education authority notification is mandatory by the age of 2 years and up to the age of 19 years.

Once the registration formalities have been completed social services are responsible for ensuring that the person is made aware of the benefits and services available to them from the various local authority departments and appropriate local or national voluntary agencies. This should preferably be done by a home visit from a social worker as part of an individual assessment and rehabilitation programme.

The statutory provisions following registration comprise central government services relating to finance and employment, and local authority provision covering daily living skills, communication and mobility training, and recreational and social activities.

Provision, particularly in the financial and employment spheres, is complex and liable to change with each budget and Social Security regulation amendment. The current situation is discussed in detail in Appendix 2. At the present time the majority of financial benefits apply only to those eligible for full blind registration. On the other hand employment and local authority social and domestic provisions may be of assistance both to registered blind and partially sighted people.

All aspects of local authority activity are constrained by limited resources. There is naturally a wide variation in the priority afforded to facilities and support services for the visually impaired. Social service departments are generally understaffed and specialist social workers are in very short supply. A RNIB survey in 1985 found ratios of client:specialist staff varying between 150:1 and over 1000:1.

In some areas a person can expect to wait many months after registration before receiving information or a visit from a social worker. In other areas, joint initiatives between Hospital Eye Service (HES) optometrists, social workers, voluntary agencies and occupational therapists have resulted in the provision of a much more rapid and efficient information and support system for newly registered people.

Overall however, there is a serious shortfall between the needs of the increasing number of visually impaired people (especially among the elderly population) and the resources and specialist help available to meet that need.

1.5   Low Vision Aid (LVA) provision

Within the NHS optical LVAs in Britain are supplied through the Hospital Eye Service, on a loan basis, without charge to the patient. The system varies a little in different health districts but in general a person will be assessed in a specialist LVA clinic following examination in the ophthalmology department or possibly as a result of a direct referral by a GP.

It is not necessary to be registered blind or partially sighted to be eligible for LVAs. It is however necessary that the person be a current eye department patient, or at least to have been assessed in the not-to-distant past. One cannot walk in 'off the street' and ask to look at magnifiers!

The majority of clinics are run by hospital based optometrists, sometimes in association with voluntary organisations such as the Partially Sighted Society, or with university optometry teaching departments. In the absence of a convenient clinic an ophthalmologist may issue authorisation for a patient to consult a local GOS (General Ophthalmic Services) optometrist who will carry out the assessment and prescribe the LVA on behalf of the hospital.

Since all units are supplied on a loan basis they remain the property of the issuing hospital/health authority. The patient retains them for as long as they are of use. Should the eye condition or the patient's visual requirements change they should be returned. The patient is then reassessed and more appropriate aids are issued as necessary.

There is a steadily increasing demand for low vision aid assessment and advice for visually handicapped people and a shortage of people able to provide such a service.

Visual handicap in the developed world is largely an age-related problem. The

Table 1.1 Estimated prevalence of major eye disease in elderly individuals in UK.

	Age group		
Condition	52–64 (%)	65–75 (%)	75–85 (%)
Glaucoma	1	2	3
Diabetic retinopathy	1	1	2
Macular degeneration	2	11	28
Cataract	5	18	45
No obvious eye disease	91	68	22

From Medical Research Council Report: Diseases of the Eye
(MRC, 1983); After Marshall, 1985.

increasing proportion of elderly people within the population will inevitably lead
to an increasing number of people with vision problems (see Fig. 1.3 and
Table 1.1). The ability to read one's own correspondence, bills, bank statements,
etc. (even somewhat laboriously with the aid of a magnifying unit) may well be a
key factor in enabling a person to retain his or her independence (Fig. 1.4). We
are dealing with a growth area!

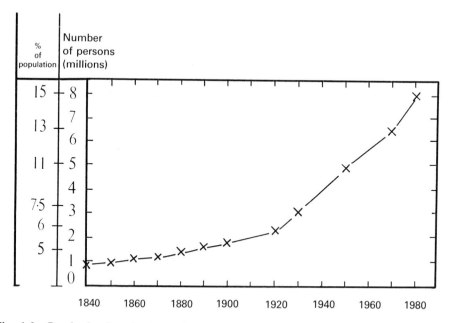

Fig. 1.3 Graph showing the increasing population in Britain, over the age of 65 years,
1840–1980. Figures presented in numerical terms (millions) and as a percentage of the
total population. Information from the Department of Population Census and Survey (*after*
Marshall, 1985).

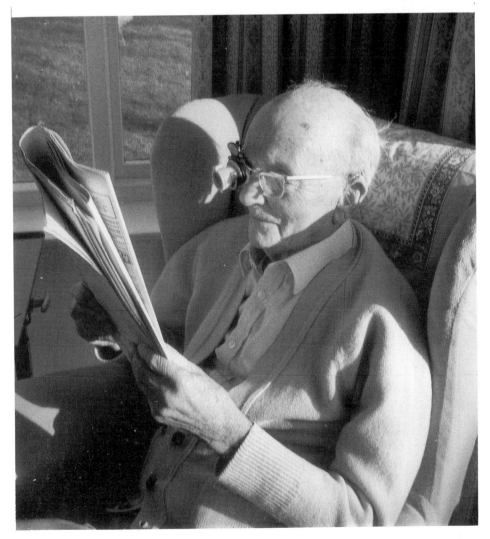

Fig. 1.4 Keeler Multicap unit (ref. 51) in use.

Improvements in the medical treatment of diabetes and other systemic diseases are leading to increased need for help for people still within the working population who require aids to enable them to continue their occupation, Fig. 1.5.

Furthermore a huge change has occurred comparatively recently in the management of blind and visually handicapped children. Before the Second World War such children were actively discouraged from using their eyes. This view is now totally discredited. Even very severely handicapped children are encouraged to make the maximum possible use of their vision. Whatever type of education

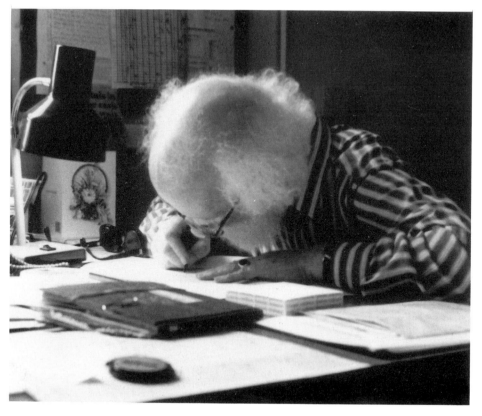

Fig. 1.5 Keeler LVA 12, bifocal spectacles, with supplementary local lighting, in use by ty-neg albino teacher (see Chapter 11, Case 5).

is involved − in special schools or integrated into mainstream schools − the aim is to enable them, wherever possible, to learn by sighted methods. Good optical assessment and provision is essential if this aim is to be achieved (Fig. 1.6).

Historically in Britain GOS optometrists have had little involvement in LVA work. A major reason has been the restrictive nature of the Department of Health regulations. NHS supply of optical aids has been channelled predominantly through clinics in the larger eye units staffed by hospital based optometrists or dispensing opticians. Encouragingly now there is a heightened awareness among all those concerned with the visually handicapped, and most importantly, ophthalmologists themselves, of the potential and scope of magnifiers and other optical aids.

Large areas of the country do not have easy access to centralised hospital-based clinics. Self-selection by the patient from a random assortment of magnifiers, or the restrictive supply of units only from one manufacturer's range, while arguably better than nothing at all, are satisfactory neither for the patient

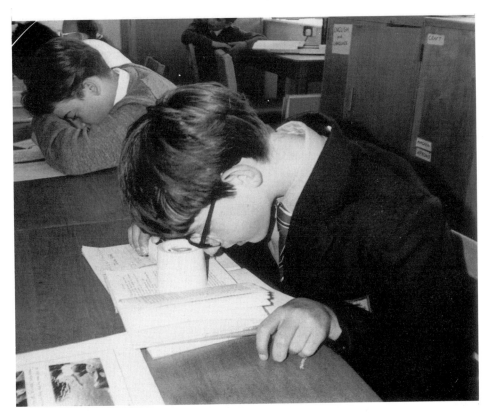

Fig. 1.6 Illuminated stand magnifier in use by a pupil at Exhall Grange School, Coventry.

from a clinical viewpoint, nor financially satisfactory for the Authority funding the service.

Ophthalmologists aware of the benefit to patients of a thorough low vision aid evaluation are increasingly looking to establish local assessment facilities. The GOS optometrist in practice is the ideal person to provide such a service in the local community. It is much more advantageous to the patient to have the LVA assessment integrated with accurate refractive measurements, since the provision of spectacles is often part of the complete 'package' of aids required.

Department of Health regulations are illogical, unfair and discriminatory in providing for the free loan of units through the HES (Hospital Eye Service), while preventing Income Support vouchers from being used to offset the cost of magnifiers supplied through the GOS.

While this is undoubtedly a major problem within the GOS in some instances, not all elderly people are in financially straitened circumstances. The fact that one has to put a price on a magnifier should not be used as a blanket excuse for ignoring its existence! In reality, the cost of many hand and stand lenses compares very favourably with 'budget' reading spectacles, and even telescopic units cost less than many top-of-the-range fashion frames.

If, however, there are circumstances in which the provision of a magnifier unit which would be of significant benefit to the patient is blocked on financial grounds, an informed but tactful approach to the GP plus social services and/or local ophthalmologist may well produce positive results.

There are large numbers of, predominantly elderly, people experiencing comparatively mild degrees of visual impairment below the 'hospital referral'/partial sight registration levels. Many such people would be helped by the provision of a simple magnifier to supplement their spectacles for specific activities. Almost all would gain enormous benefit from advice and instruction in lighting use, colour contrast, availability of large print facilities and so on.

Individual optometrists are likely to need to take the initiative and make their interest known to local GPs, ophthalmologists and social service departments. Since optometrists already have the knowledge of optics, pathology and the visual process which forms the basis of all visual assessment, only a modest amount of additional detailed specialist information is necessary in order that partial sight assessment, advice and management can become a rewarding, sometimes frustrating, but always interesting extension of normal professional activity.

Questions

1. What is the reference number of the form used for blind/partial sight registration purposes

    (a)   In England and Wales?
    (b)   In Scotland?

    (See section [1.3].)

2. Who makes the legal decision regarding registration?
    (See section [1.3].)

3. Summarise the visual criteria for:

    (a)   full blind registration, and
    (b)   partial sight registration.

    (See section [1.3].)

4. What happens to the registration document after it has been completed?
    (See section [1.4].)

5. Who is responsible for ensuring that people are made aware of their statutory rights following registration?
    (See section [1.4].)

6. What are the financial benefits conditional upon blind registration?
    (See Appendix 2.)

7. What are the major causes of visual disability in Britain?
    (See section [1.5].)

8. How are low vision aids supplied and funded through the NHS?
    (See section [1.5].)

CHAPTER 2

A Summary of the Commoner Causes of Visual Impairment

2.1 Summary notes on basic genetics
(McKusick, 1968; Waardenburg *et al.*, 1961)

Normal individuals have 23 pairs of chromosomes. The first 22 pairs, known as autosomal chromosomes, are identical in shape, i.e. homologous. The 23rd pair are the sex chromosomes, labelled X (female) and Y (male). These are very different to each other in shape, i.e. non-homologous. Genes are located segmentially along the length of the chromosome. Pairs of genes which control the same trait occupy the same locus (that is — are situated opposite each other) on pairs of homologous chromosomes. Such pairs of genes are said to be allelic.

Accurate genetic counselling depends on being able to distinguish between the three general modes of inheritance:

- many genes interacting to produce one trait, e.g. refractive error;
- one gene influencing the formation of many traits, e.g. Marfan's syndrome; Laurence—Moon—Biedl syndrome;
- one gene producing one trait.

The classic modes of transmission can usually be applied only to this last group.

2.1.1 Autosomal genes

These are not sex-linked, thus characteristics they control have an equal possibility of occurrence in males and females.

Autosomal recessive

Genes mediating a given trait are either 'normal' or 'abnormal', with no intermediate forms. The normal gene is dominant to the abnormal gene such that an abnormal trait is only manifest in individuals who inherit an abnormal gene from both parents.

The recessive nature of the abnormal gene means that it frequently passes

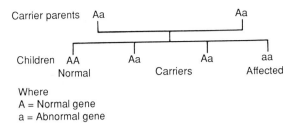

Fig. 2.1 Autosomal recessive inheritance.

down through generations without its presence being suspected until a child is born with the particular condition. Thereafter there is a one in four chance of other children within the family being affected, with a one in two chance of a child being a carrier.

Consanguinity between parents, or marriages between people from within comparatively, localised communities significantly increase the likelihood of recessive traits becoming manifest.

Autosomal dominant

This is the situation where the abnormal gene is dominant and expresses itself even in the presence of its normal allele. Any individual inheriting the dominant abnormal gene will manifest signs of the disorder and carries a one in two chance of passing the defect onto any child.

Unlike recessive conditions dominant traits show a broad range of severity or penetrance. Affected individuals within the same family can differ markedly in the severity of the abnormal characteristic.

2.1.2   Sex-linked transmission (X-linked)

The Y chromosome carries only genes concerned with male traits and has no genes allelic to those on the paired X-chromosome. However, the longer X-chromosome carries genes controlling many general traits in addition to those mediating female characteristics. Sex-linked inherited eye condition must therefore always relate to the X-chromosome.

Recessive X-linked

Characterised by unaffected female carriers of a condition which is normally only manifest in male children (e.g. red–green colour deficiency, ocular albinism).

Normally, sons have a one in two chance of being affected and daughters have a one in two chance of being carriers. It is possible, although statistically rare,

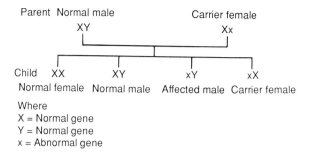

Fig. 2.2 Common form of X-linked recessive inheritance.

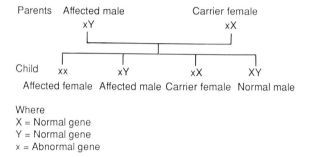

Fig. 2.3 Statistically rare recessive X-linked inheritance giving rise to an affected female.

for a female to be affected by a recessive X-linked condition. She would need to have a father affected by the condition and a mother who is a carrier.

Dominant X-linked

A large family tree covering three or more generations is necessary to differentiate between dominant X-linked and dominant autosomal inheritance patterns. If limited information is available on only two generations, it is normally impossible to separate the two options. The transmission pattern is similar in both instances in the case of affected females. However, a male affected by a dominant X-linked condition can only pass the defective gene to female children; unlike the autosomal dominant situation, in which the condition is passed equally to male and female children.

2.2   Conditions affecting children

The majority of visual problems among young children result from congenital defects. Many, although by no means all, such defects are genetically determined. Most regions have specialist genetic counselling clinics to which ophthalmologists and paediatricians can refer families for detailed guidance. It would be most inadvisable for an optometrist to become involved in detailed predictions in any particular individual case. On the other hand, it is very helpful to be aware of any genetic influences affecting the eye conditions encountered in LVA work.

Such genetic factors, likely prognosis and rate of change influence the frequency of examination. Such background knowledge enables one to give more constructive advice, guidance and support to parents or teachers who are endeavouring to 'do their best' on behalf of the visually impaired child.

The majority of structural defects are non-progressive. Vision will depend entirely on the site and extent of the abnormality. In general the visual performance of the child improves with increasing maturity. It is very much influenced by parental and environmental factors, but frequently achievements and functional abilities belie the distance acuity measurements. It should also be remembered that a great many visually impaired children have comparatively normal peripheral fields and plentiful accommodation.

The following notes are intended to provide a summary of the major factors relating to the commoner causes of visual impairment. The various conditions reviewed are grouped broadly in age-related categories.

2.2.1 Nystagmus

Nystagmus may occur without any other evidence of ocular pathology – congenital idiopathic nystagmus – or in association with any other congenital ocular defect. Visual acuity is related to the amplitude of movement, superimposed, where appropriate, on any additional pathological effects.

Nystagmus increases on dissociation and with stress, and reduces on accommodation. It is a non-progressive condition which appears marginally to improve with age. Inheritance of congenital idiopathic nystagmus can be (Duke Elder, 1964):

(1)   most common: X-linked dominant;
(2)   fairly frequent: X-linked recessive;
(3)   rare: autosomal dominant and autosomal recessive.

2.2.2 Albinism

Total oculocutaneous albinism

The incidence of this condition is approximately 1 in 20 000 of the population. It is due to an absence of enzyme tyrosinase, which converts an intermediate product of protein metabolism into melanin.

Inheritance: autosomal recessive.

The condition is characterised by pink/red pupils, rapid nystagmus, photo-phobia, reduced VA, orange/red fundus with choroidal vessels visible, absence of macular reflex resulting from a failure of foveal differentiation. Dark adaptation and colour vision are normal.

Oculocutaneous albinism is subdivided into two types which may be differen-tiated in infancy by biochemical tests on hair follicles.

Tyrosinase-positive (ty-pos) group: This is the milder form, with albinism very marked at birth with pigmentation increasing very slowly with age, mainly at pupil margin of iris. The iris transilluminates markedly in Europeans, but not in Asian or African races. There is a mild-severe nystagmus and reduced acuity which does improve slowly with age.

Tyrosinase-negative (ty-neg) group: Blue-grey iris which transilluminates in all races. Severe nystagmus with markedly reduced VA (3/60−6/60) which does not improve with age.

Ty-pos and ty-neg forms of total albinism are non-allelic (Trevor Roper, 1952). Two parents with total albinism, one of each type, will thus produce normally pigmented children.

Partial albinism

This is felt to result from a functional insufficiency or defective distribution of the tyrosinase enzyme system throughout the body. Carriers of autosomal recessive albinism show no ocular signs of abnormality.

Ocular albinism

This is a form of incomplete albinism, characterised by a deficiency of pigment in the retinal pigment epithelium.

Inheritance: X-linked recessive; carrier mother, affected male children.

Superficial ocular appearance will depend on underlying racial group involved, varying from light blue to brown. There will be mild nystagmus, but variable iris transillumination and fundus depigmentation. Diagnosis often depends on examination of the mother. Female carriers of X-linked ocular albinism show irregular areas of iris transillumination and scattered patches of depigmentation in the fundus.

Ocular albinism tends to improve with age with a slowly increasing level of general ocular, hair and skin pigmentation. Acuity typically in the 6/12 to 6/36 range.

2.2.3 Micropthalmos ('small eye')

This may be pure micropthalmos (nanophthalmos) a small, but otherwise normal eye; or complicated micropthalmos, when the small globe is associated with colobomas or other developmental abnormalities.

Micropthalmos is usually, but not invariably, associated with high hypermetropia, nystagmus and a subnormal acuity. Such eyes have a shallow anterior chamber and frequently develop glaucoma.

Inheritance: autosomal recessive or autosomal dominant with low penetrance; or sporadic.

2.2.4 Bupthalmos (congenital glaucoma)

Elevated intraocular pressure (IOP) resulting from developmental abnormalities obstructing drainage. It is manifest shortly after birth. Two thirds of cases are bilateral; the eyes are generally myopic with an enlarged globe and cornea, with varying degrees of corneal opacity, disruption to Descemet's membrane, corneal endothelium and neuroretina.

Prognosis is improving but is still problematical. Much depends on the time of onset (therefore on the extent of the structural anomaly) and on prompt diagnosis and treatment. Repeated surgery may be required.

Inheritance: majority sporadic; a few autosomal recessive.

2.2.5 Aniridia

The absence of iris is generally associated with photophobia, nystagmus and abnormal foveal differentiation. Moderate/high refractive errors are common. The condition is stationary unless structural abnormality in the trabecular region induces glaucoma. Associated malformation in the ciliary body may give rise to accommodative problems.

Inheritance: strongly autosomal dominant.

2.2.6 Congenital cataracts

Duke Elder (1964) defines a congenital cataract as being opacity in the foetal or innermost part of the infantile nucleus. Within that general classification one may encounter wide variation in opacity appearance and size. There is also a wide variation in the aetiology of the failure of normal development giving rise to the cataract.

(a) *Genetic factors*: autosomal dominant with variable penetrance.

> Anterior polar cataracts: usually small, stationary, little interference with vision.
> Posterior polar cataracts: occur in a stationary, delineated form, or as a diffuse, cortical opacity which progresses after birth.
> Central nuclear cataracts: approx 25% of all congenital cataracts (Fig. 2.4(a)).
> Lamellar cataracts, often with 'riders', where the opacity effects one lamella of the fibres surrounding the nucleus, anteriorly and posteriorly (Fig. 2.4(b)).

All genetically determined congenital cataracts, although varying in size and density are characterised by their central position surrounded by clear cortex.

(b) *Metabolic factors*: congenital cataracts are known to result from disturbance to many systemic chemical processes. Disruption or imbalance of endocrine system, calcium metabolism and carbohydrate metabolism (e.g. mother with diabetes) can all result in generalised lenticular opacity.

(c) *Toxic/infectious factors*: the commonest and most widely known agent in this category is infection with rubella virus in the first trimester of pregnancy. Cataract is frequently associated with severely impaired hearing, a heart defect and possibly mental retardation.

(d) *Trauma*:
Surgical intervention in cases of bilateral congenital cataract will depend on the severity of the problem. The near vision implication occasioned by the loss of accommodation should be considered particularly carefully. A severe uniocular cataract presents an even greater management problem. The long term visual result is problematical even if surgery is undertaken and an extended-wear contact lens is fitted at a very early age.

Frequent refractive assessment of aphakic children is vital since the level of hypermetropia drops quite rapidly as the eye develops during the first few years of life.

2.2.7   Marfan's Syndrome

A connective tissue disease affecting the eye, skeleton and cardiovascular system. Ocular effects are of displaced lenses with defective zonular fibres. These frequently give rise to high levels of myopia and astigmatism. If lens displacement is marked, refraction should be carried out through both the phakic and aphakic pupil areas, prescribing the alternative which gives rise to better acuity.

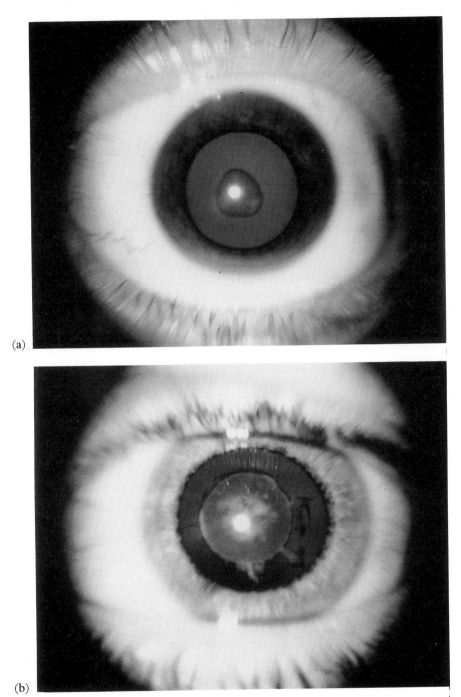

Fig. 2.4 (a) Congenital nuclear cataract; (b) Congenital lamellar cataract with 'riders'. Both photographed through dilated pupils.

A gradual weakening of the zonular fibres may cause increasing lens displacement and a tendency for the lens to vibrate with sudden eye movements. Both effects obviously lead to increasing visual disruption.

Skeletal effects are abnormally long fingers, toes and limb bones so that children are significantly taller and thinner than normal.

Inheritance: autosomal dominant.

2.2.8   High myopia

Myopia is relatively unusual among infants in general. Atkinson & Braddick (1984) on a photorefractive study of over 1000 infants, aged 6−9 months, found 4.5% to be myopic below 3D and only 0.5% myopia greater than 3D. Myopia is much more common among premature infants (16%) and approximately half of all babies with retinopathy of prematurity (retrolental fibroplasia) have been found to be myopic (Nissenhorn *et al.*, 1983).

High myopia is associated with a larger than normal globe, large pale discs, peripapillary atrophy, scleral crescent and thin neuroretina. The incidence of retinal detachment is high. Parents of highly myopic children should be warned to take any report of sudden floaters or visual disturbance seriously and to have the child checked urgently.

In the longer term, highly myopic eyes are prone to macular changes, often accompanied by deep retinal or sub-retinal haemorrhages (Foster-Fuch's Spot), or splits in Brüch's membrane.

2.2.9   Coloboma

Coloboma is caused by faulty closure of the embryonic fissure around the 4th−5th week of pregnancy. A coloboma may be partial or complete. It may vary from as little as a notch in the iris margin to a large abnormality involving disc, retina, choroid, ciliary body, iris and possibly the lens.

Extensive colobomas are commonly associated with nystagmus, strabismus and micropthalmos. Acuity naturally depends on the extent and position of the coloboma.

Inheritance: usually spontaneous; occasionally autosomal dominant.

2.2.10   Achromatopsia

Achromatopsia, congenital cone dysfunction or rod monochromatism gives rise to monochromatic vision which may be almost normal in very dim light, but grey, with variations in relative luminous efficiency, in daylight.

It is always associated with marked pathological changes. Central acuity is severely reduced; nystagmus and extreme photophobia are always evident and there may be a central scotoma.

Inheritance: 70% autosomal recessive; rest unknown origin.

2.3   Older children and adult working population

2.3.1   Corneal dystrophy

Corneal disturbance can result from a multitude of causes; inherited, infectious, acquired, metabolic and traumatic. In the developing world corneal disease associated with protein and vitamin A deficiency is a major cause of blindness.

Corneal dystrophies, although primarily related to one level, may sometimes cause pathological changes throughout the whole corneal structure.

- Epithelial, e.g. Meesman's dystrophy (dominant).
- Stromal, e.g. granular and lattice dystrophies (dominant) and macular dystrophy (recessive).
- Endothelial, e.g. Fuch's dystrophy (dominant).

Corneal problems tend to blur vision without introducing any specific visual field abnormalities. Glare may be a significant problem depending on the distribution and density of the opacity. Age of onset and rate of progression is likewise enormously variable.

Keratoconus is generally included in any list of corneal dystrophies, although happily modern contact lens technique and advances in surgical keratoplasty have removed most sufferers from the partially sighted ranks. The condition has noticeable associations with asthma and atopic skin problems and usually presents as increasing myopic astigmatism in teenage patients. Ultimately the majority of cases are bilateral although one eye tends to be more severely affected than the other.

2.3.2   Juvenile macular dystrophy
   (Michaelson, 1980)

There are a number of primary, heredo-macular dystrophies which probably all belong within the same general clinical groups. Familial characteristics are usually maintained in that all members of a family with the condition are approximately alike in age of onset, rate of progression and general evolution.

All are bilateral macular degenerations with no central nervous system involvement. Onset has a preference for times when physiological stress is most marked; birth, 6−8 years (second dentition), 12−15 years (puberty), and at the end of normal growth (20 years). Ophthalmoscopic appearance varies from fine pigmentary disturbance to macular holes, haemorrhages, colloid and exudate (Duke Elder, 1967).

Vitelliform macular degeneration – Best's disease

This is a dominantly inherited disorder, manifest congenitally or early in life as a round/oral, raised, well delineated lesion, 1–4 disc diameters in size, centred on the macula. It is yellowish in colour (like egg yolk). Visual acuity is good at first but deteriorates later as the original lesion absorbs to leave a rounded, atrophic, pigmented scarred area. Colour vision and EOG (electro-oculogram) are significantly abnormal even in early stages of the disease. Dark adaptation, peripheral fields and the ERG (electro-retinogram) are normal.

Stargardt's disease

Stargardt's disease is a term applied rather loosely to macular disorders which appear to be a primary degeneration of the retinal elements of the fovea, manifest roughly between the ages of 8–20 years.

There may be little to see ophthalmoscopically at first, which unfortunately sometimes results in the child's complaints being dismissed as malingering. Visual acuity declines, colour vision defects start to appear, and the child may experience difficulty in bright light. The macular reflex distorts and is then lost, as abnormal pigmentation appears at both maculae. There are often prominent yellowish flecks in the macular and posterior polar areas.

Visual loss progresses gradually, but is generally well established by the age of 30 years, with final VA 1/60–6/60. The red–green colour defect progresses towards achromatopsia. Dark adaptation and peripheral fields remain normal. *Inheritance pattern*: normally autosomal recessive, although dominant and sporadic instances have been documented. Fundal appearances are similar between affected members of the same family, but differ considerably in different families.

Fundus flavimaculatus

This is a condition characterised by a large number of yellowish lesions/flecks throughout the posterior pole and/or equator of the retina. These flecks are probably pigment epithelial defects, and may be associated in due course with atrophic macular degeneration. Visual defects vary from slight to severe, depending on the degree of macular involvement.

Stargardt's disease is often considered to be a form of fundus flavimaculatus (Krill & Deutman, 1972). Other authorities differentiate the two conditions by the time of onset of the macular involvement. The macula is affected early in Stargardt's disease, but not until a later stage (if at all) in flavimaculatus (Michaelson, 1980).

Bull's eye dystrophy – cone degenerations

Another condition, dominant or recessive inheritance or sporadic in nature, in which visual loss often precedes ophthalmoscopic signs. The macular region eventually assumes a characteristic 'bull's eye' appearance of a sharply defined ring of depigmentation surrounding a central homogenous dark red area. Visual effects and prognosis are very variable.

2.3.3   Retinitis pigmentosa (RP)

A primary tapetoretinal degeneration, producing dystrophy of the neuro-epithelium, and atrophy and loss of the retinal internal limiting membrane. It initially affects rods in the equatorial region.

Signs are typically night blindness, difficulty with sudden changes in illumination, and annular scotoma in the mid-periphery 30–50° from fixation which later spreads both towards the periphery and towards fixation involving cones. Field defect eventually becomes a generalised constriction leading to the typical RP tunnel vision effect.

Ophthalmoscopic appearance is of bone corpuscle pigmentary deposits along the vessels, attenuated retinal arteries and a secondary 'waxy' optic atrophy. Posterior sub-capsular cataracts may occur as a late feature of RP. There is macular sparing until a comparatively late stage of the disease.

Inheritance patterns are mixed (Klein *et al.*, 1967): 90% autosomal recessive (with a relatively high incidence of consanguinity), 9% autosomal dominant, 1% sex-linked recessive.

The aetiology and major biochemical defect in RP is still unknown and there is no effective treatment. Night blindness is generally evident in childhood, with retinal changes becoming evident in early teens. The condition, although always progressive, is very variable. Central vision is typically lost in the patient's fifties.

EOG and dark adaption measurements are abnormal at a very early stage.

RP may occur as part of a more generalised syndrome. Usher's Syndrome – congenital, non-progressive hearing loss combined with RP occurring in childhood. Lawrence–Moon–Biedl Syndrome – RP, polydactyly, obesity, hypogonadism and mental retardation.

2.3.4   Diabetes

Diabetic eye disease involves progressive changes caused by disruption of arteriolar blood flow and structure of the capillary vessel walls. Microaneurisms, blot haemorrhages, hard and soft 'cotton wool' exudates comprise the characteristic diabetic retinopathy appearance, either generally throughout the retina or centred on the posterior pole as a diabetic maculopathy.

Increasing severity of the disease produces new vessel formation, associated with areas of capillary closure and ischaemia. This proliferative stage carries a high risk of more extensive retinal and vitreous haemorrhage, vitreous traction and severe visual loss. Two thirds of patients with proliferative retinopathy also have rubeosis irides and associated glaucoma.

Primary open angle glaucoma is reported to be three times more frequent among adult diabetics than non-diabetics (Armstrong *et al.*, 1960).

Quoted figures vary, but as a general guide, it is found that 2% of all diabetics are blind from diabetic retinopathy. It is the most important systemic cause of blindness and the commonest cause of blindness in the 40−60 year age group.

Incidence of retinopathy varies with the duration and age of onset of the diabetes. After 15 years, approximately 50% Type I (insulin dependent, juvenile onset) diabetics show signs of mild background retinopathy, of which some 10% have more severe proliferative changes. Significant retinopathy is very rare among Type I diabetics until the disease is of approximately 12 years' duration.

Good diabetic control is a significant factor in delaying the onset and severity of the retinopathy for Type I diabetics.

Type II (non-insulin dependent, maturity onset) diabetics may develop significant retinopathy earlier (5−10 years' duration). After a similar 15 year period, 75% will have a noticeable level of background retinopathy, with 15% suffering proliferative disease. Many Type II diabetics have an established retinopathy when the disease is first discovered, which may not resolve or improve materially even when good diabetic control is achieved.

Laser photocoagulation can be helpful in some cases of diabetic maculopathy. Ablation of retinal areas affected either by capilliary leakage or ischaemia from capillary shut down, reduces retinopathy and induces regression of the abnormal new vessels.

Diabetic patients frequently suffer from glare from media opacities. They are likely to have patchy field defects, and colour vision and contrast sensitivity abnormalities. Variation in blood sugar levels can also give rise to refractive power fluctuation. The complexity and variability of the disease process often results in frequent assessment and reassessment of diabetic LVA patients.

2.4   Elderly age group

The incidence of many systemic and specifically ocular problems increases with age, so will obviously occur with more frequency among a cross section of elderly visually impaired patients, although most may be found occasionally among younger people.

Ocular degenerative conditions, such as Fuch's and other corneal dystrophies, myopic degeneration, chorioretinal atrophy, etc., will tend to increase in severity with increasing age. There will be a greater incidence of vascular disorders, artery and vein occlusions, visual field loss from brain haemorrhages, cerebral tumours and so on.

Happily, improved surgical techniques and pharmacological therapeutic control are steadily reducing the number of people suffering severe visual loss from glaucoma and senile cataract.

The greatest cause of visual disability in the developed world is senile macular degeneration. Thus the major consumer of low vision aid services is the elderly person afflicted by this problem.

2.4.1 Age related or senile macular degeneration (SMD)

SMD is a complex condition involving histological changes in the choriocapillaris, Brüch's membrane and the retinal pigment epithelium. These structures are so closely associated with each other that a loss of function in one tissue will upset the function and physical structure of the other tissues.

Much research effort is being concentrated in this area. The condition is generally bilateral, although the second eye may not be affected for many years after central vision has been lost in the first eye.

The early stage is characterised by fine pigment stippling and loss of reflex at the macula. More extensive pigmentary disturbance, white/yellow colloid bodies or drusen may develop with initially minimal visual loss.

The chronic, slowly progressive, dry, atrophic form of SMD is not amenable to any treatment. On the other hand, if patients with macular drusen experience any sudden onset visual distortion, this suggests they are progressing to the haemorrhagic, disciform stage of the disease. They should be referred urgently for ophthalmological assessment.

Results are very mixed, but some oedematous, haemorrhagic disciform lesions benefit from laser photocoagulation. For treatment to be attempted, the site of the leaking, neovascular membrane (identified by fluorescein angiography) must be paramacular, and preferably temporal to the fovea. Laser treatment in the vicinity of the fovea obviously requires a high degree of patient co-operation and extreme accuracy and care on the part of the ophthalmologist! The aim is to seal off the leaking abnormal vessels, and to prevent further fluid seeping into the macula area.

Patients with SMD will have varying degrees of central scotoma, visual acuity and colour vision loss. Peripheral fields remain normal and it is important to stress to such patients that 'edge vision' will always be retained. The person will thus always have reasonable mobility and should be able to maintain a fairly independent lifestyle.

Questions

1 Many ocular disorders are genetically determined. Give an example of an autosomal recessive condition. How would you explain the inheritance pattern to a patient? What is the likelihood of an affected person passing the condition onto a child?
   (See section [2.1.1].)

2. Can a man, affected by a X-linked disorder, transmit the disorder to his son?
    (See section [2.1.2].)

3. What are the causes of congenital cataract? How would you differentiate a genetically determined cataract from a cataract due to other causes?
    (See section [2.2.6].)

4. Describe the various forms of albinism.
    (See section [2.2.2].)

5. What is the incidence of myopia among:

    (a)   full term infants?
    (b)   premature infants?

    (See section [2.2.8].)

6. Outline the characteristics of the various types of juvenile macular degeneration.
    (See section [2.3.2].)

7. What are the early sign and diagnostic features of retinitis pigmentosa?
    (See section [2.3.3].)

8. Name the two syndromes which feature retinitis pigmentosa.
    (See section [2.3.3].)

9. Diabetes is the commonest cause of blindness in the 40−60 year age group. How does the incidence and severity of retinopathy vary between Type I and Type II diabetics?
    (See section [2.3.4].)

10. Differentiate the two different forms of senile macular degeneration. Which form may sometimes benefit from laser treatment? How urgent is the referral?
(See section [2.4].)

CHAPTER 3

Refractive Examination Routine for a Visually Impaired Patient

3.1   Adult patient

Many people attend an LVA assessment accompanied by a friend or relative. It is often preferable however, to conduct the initial 'history and symptoms' and refractive examination with the person alone.

It is not uncommon for patients to disguise the full extent of their problems from family and friends. A desire 'not to be a burden', or a fear of losing independence, or a job if the true extent of the problem were known may cause the person to play down and understate the visual difficulties. The practitioner is more likely to get a true assessment if the patient is satisfied that the information provided will be treated in confidence.

Towards the end of the assessment, when the patient is being instructed in the use of specific aids and the conversation has become more general in nature, it is very helpful if the friend/relative can be brought into the room to listen. Two people listening to advice and instruction on lighting, non-optical aids and ways of improving visibility, etc., is much to be preferred than the patient listening alone. Far more will be remembered and hopefully put into practice once the person is back at home.

3.1.1   Preliminary discussion:
expanded history and symptoms

In principle the information that the optometrist is seeking to elicit from a visually impaired patient is similar to that established in a normal patient's 'history and symptoms' conversation. Certain areas require more detailed investigation but one should not neglect the standard routine questions.

A suggested pattern might be as follows:

(1) *General questions*:
- General health?
- Headaches?
- Use of any systemic medication?

30

- Use of any ocular medication?
- Any relevant family ocular or general health problems?
- Any hearing difficulty?

(2) *Questions relating to the specific ocular condition*:
- Onset: how long has the eye problem existed?
- Progress: how rapidly has it changed?
- What investigations have been carried out?

> e.g.:   Ophthalmoscopy only?
> Visual field assessment?
> Orthoptic investigation?
> Colour vision tests?
> Photographic or fluorescein angiography investigation?
> Electrodiagnostic or neurological investigations?

- What treatment has been received?

> e.g.:   Drug therapy?
> Surgery?
> Laser treatment?

- What does the person know about the ocular and vision problems?
- What is believed to be the likely prognosis?
- Is any further treatment being considered?
- Is the person still an active hospital patient? When were they: last seen/ next appointment/discharged?
- Has a full blind or partial sight registration been done?
- Any previous experience of optical aids? If so, what type?

(3) *Functional questions: specifically how does the visual problem affect their life?*
General mobility and independence:
- How did the person travel to this appointment?
- Is it possible to cope with traffic and crossing roads alone?
- In general, will they go out and travel unaided?
- Is there an awareness of any particular field defect?
- Are steps, kerbs and other street furniture a problem – no difficulty or bumping into lamp-posts and so on?
- Is there a need to read bus numbers, notice boards, time-tables, etc.?
- Any problems when shopping? Reading prices? Differentiating coins and banknotes?

Light and colour:

- How does light affect the person's sight?

- Is vision subjectively better on bright sunny days, overcast days or in the dark?
- How are colours seen? Not very well/all about equally/some colours more easily seen than others?

Acuity at home:

- Is it possible to make sense of the television picture? In colour or black and white?
- Is vision adequate to read letters and sign documents?
- What type of material is read now and for how long?
- Would the person like to be able to read more extensively? What type of material — books, newspapers, knitting patterns, crosswords, etc.?
- Are there any problems with the numbers on the telephone dial?
- Are there any problems in the kitchen? Preparing food? Reading cooker dials?
- Have any particular hobbies or activities had to be curtailed? Sewing, music, gardening, sport, bingo, etc.?
- What sort of lighting is available at home?

Occupational or educational requirements:

- What is the nature of the job?
- Size and working distance of task details?
- Light levels and availability of local lighting?
- Attitudes of employer and colleagues?

If at school:

- Is the person integrated into a mainstream school or in a special unit of some kind?
- Is it necessary to work from the blackboard? Can they manage, and if not, what happens now?
- What about sport, laboratory and practical subjects?
- Are photocopier enlarger facilities available?
- Attitudes of school staff?

(4) *Social considerations*:
- Does the person live alone or with family?
- In general terms, how does the person occupy the day?
  Predominantly alone or pursuing an active social life?
- Are there any other medical problems which are likely to further complicate the management of the person's visual problem? Such things as deafness, arthritis, Parkinsons' disease or more general manual unsteadiness or any type of mental deficiency?

- Are family and friends supportive? Would they help the patient to practice with an optical aid or are they overprotective or negative in their attitude?
- Are there any major disabilities in the patient's immediate family, especially spouse, which might adversely affect the overall situation?
- Is there any social service input now? Any contact with a social worker? Meals-on-wheels? Home help, etc.?

(5) *General discussion*:

During the course of this detailed 'history and symptoms' discussion the practitioner will have built up a picture of the individual and problems covering all aspects of the person's life. Some points, such as job requirements for example, will be returned to and considered in much greater detail at a later stage in conjunction with provision of specific aids. Nontheless some reference does need to be made to them within this initial phase of the assessment in the interests of obtaining a balanced view of the person's situation.

Regrettably, in the absence of a magic wand we cannot tackle all problems – or not in a single assessment anyway! It is therefore necessary to establish what each person feels to be their major problem areas. What do they miss most of all? What would they most like to be able to do or do again?

This leads onto a final very important question which must be considered if disappointment and misunderstanding are to be avoided, namely 'what do you think I can do for you?'

Patients can harbour quite unrealistic expectations of a LVA assessment. Despite what they have been told by their doctors, sometimes even despite being registered blind, many cling to the hope that somewhere the 'magic wand' does exist and that a 'stronger pair of glasses' will somehow transform the situation and restore their vision to normal.

They may have received a full explanation of their eye condition from their ophthalmologist, but the noise and bustle of an average hospital out-patient department is not conducive to absorbing information, particularly if blind or partial sight registration is being proposed at the same time. From time to time I have been present when an ophthalmologist has given a detailed explanation of an eye problem to a patient and so I know exactly what has been said. On meeting the patient again a few weeks later for a LVA assessment I usually find they were so overwhelmed by the whole hospital 'package' that almost none of the information has been remembered at all, much less understood.

In order to make progress, it may be essential that the practitioner takes time to explain (or to re-explain!) the nature of the visual problem, clearly and in straightforward non-technical terms. Even without access to the hospital records, ophthalmoscopy plus the information obtained from the patient should enable the optometrist to make a reliable diagnosis on which to base explanations to the patient.

Cloudy, dirty windows and opaque bathroom-window type glass are easily understood analogies for corneal and lenticular problems. Most people have a reasonable basic comprehension of the workings of a camera which can be utilised to explain retinal, nerve fibre pathway and cortical problems. It is readily understood that a clear photograph requires both an accurately set-up lens systems and an unflawed film, and that a defect in the film will inevitably produce a defect in the photograph even though the lens system is correct. Link the function of the film to that of the retina and the person with macula disease for example, hopefully will grasp why a simple change of spectacles will not solve the vision problem.

The camera analogy, modified now to a television camera linked by wires to a control room, is helpful for patients struggling to understand problems of nerve fibre pathway and cortical damage. If the relative position of the damage can be visualised in terms of the nerve fibres equating to the wiring and the brain being equivalent to the control room, then the patient will be in a better position to accept the reality of the situation.

Comparison with cameras and dirty car windscreens and so on are very helpful but the practitioner must be aware of his or her own attitude when 'putting across' this type of information and should be careful not to 'talk-down' to the patient. The patient is visually impaired, not stupid. Nor, in most cases, is the patient deaf. The unconscious tendency to raise one's voice must also be firmly restrained.

Practitioners with access to medical records can obviously significantly prune the history routine in some areas. The majority of points outlined will need to be touched upon when dealing with a completely unknown patient. The skill and experience of the practitioner will determine how much time is spent on this part of the routine. Whatever approach is adopted by the practitioner he or she should endeavour to put the patient at ease. Most normal patients perform better and may appear to see more clearly when relaxed than when in a flustered apprehensive state. This is even more noticeable when assessing visually impaired people in general, and particularly significant when dealing with nystagmus. Obviously one must take account of time, but the 'history and symptoms' session should be as relaxed as possible, rather than resembling a rehearsal for *Mastermind*!

All magnification devices have severe limitations when compared with normal sight. They can only be successful if the patient adopts a positive attitude. Time spent at this stage establishing needs and helping the person towards a realistic appreciation of what is possible will contribute enormously to the ultimate successful acceptance and use of optical aids and constructive use of their residual vision.

3.1.2   Refractive routine: adult patient

(1)   Unaided vision/VA with existing R_x

Measurements should be taken monocularly and binocularly for distance and near vision. A reasonable, but not exaggerated light level should be used for the near readings. Binocular assessment is particularly important in cases of nystagmus where the acuity may drop significantly in the monocular situation as the amplitude of the nystagmus increases with dissociation.

(2)   Cover test: distance and near

Common sense and ingenuity may be required in the choice of target. Pen torches and corneal reflections can give information if all else fails! Many children with congenital ocular disorders fail to develop normal binocular function. Tropias are common. People may use one eye for distance and the other eye for near vision. Divergent deviations are often encountered among older people with acquired defects. Knowledge of the preferred fixing eye is useful at a later stage if monocular units are being considered.

(3)   Motility

The pen torch as conventionally used can be seen by all but the most severely visually impaired subjects (when it is not relevant anyway). In many instances it will be a very gross test but should nevertheless provide information as to the existence of any significant neuro-muscular abnormality. A severe limitation of ocular movement has obvious implications both for mobility and for the scanning movements normally used in reading.

(4)   Confrontation test

A full visual field examination is not usually necessary as part of a LVA assessment although it may of course be undertaken periodically to monitor the progress of the basic medical condition. However, a confrontation test may be useful to detect any gross defect which might affect mobility.

    Common sense, again should be applied to the choice of target. Those with macular lesions will respond to normal Bjerrum screen or 'hat-pin' targets. Moving fingers or a waving hand will be the order of the day for other patients.

(5)   Establishing the basic distance refraction and acuity

It is important to establish an accurate distance prescription especially with regard to cylinders. This may not appreciably improve distance VA but may be of considerable significance when near vision magnification is being considered. The basic procedure follows the standard routine of retinoscopy (if possible) and subjective assessment. A keratometry reading may sometimes be of help when confronted by an abnormal cornea and/or an impossible retinoscopy reflex! A shorter than normal retinoscopy working distance may also be beneficial.

It is essential to have a three metre and preferably an additional one metre chart available, such that the person can see something reasonably clearly right from the start. It is very demoralising to be confronted by an illuminated black and white haze! Furthermore, it is unrealistic to expect any useful subjective discrimination under such conditions. Conversely, just seeing an extra letter on a 1 m chart engenders a much more positive attitude on the part of the patient.

Normal routine is further modified by using larger than normal power changes ($\pm$1.00DS rather than $\pm$0.25DS) and a high powered cross-cyl ($\pm$1.00 or $\pm$1.50). Most important, take your time. A patient with a field defect may well have to scan or adopt an unusual head posture in order to see the chart and will frequently be slower than normal when assessing lens changes.

If the refractive power has been assessed using a 1 m chart the final R_x must be reduced by +1.00DS to render it a true distance prescription. The +0.33DS theoretical compensation necessary when using a 3 m chart is generally ignored.

Once the distance R_x has been established one should try to give the patient the opportunity of deciding whether the improvement in acuity is really of significance. Simply look out of a door or window to compare the 'real world' appearance with and without the lenses. Don't prejudge the lens effects. The permutations of pathology, plus field, plus patient psychology and experience are endless. An improvement in VA which passes unnoticed by one patient may be of immense benefit to another. Snellen measurements only relate to central vision. A patient with a sizeable refractive error and a central scotoma may show negligible improvement in central acuity but gain significant help with mobility from the improved peripheral image quality. Unfortunately this is particularly difficult to evaluate in a consulting room environment owing to the artificial restriction imposed on peripheral vision by the bulk of the trial frame and the widespread use of reduced aperture trial lenses.

Further useful information can be gained by including two additional procedures at the end of the normal subjective routine.

(6)   Pinhole VA

This is particularly useful for patients with patchy media opacities and/or corneal abnormalities.

Corneal problems giving improved pinhole VA might well justify a contact lens trial. Media opacities demonstrating improved VA through a pinhole may sometimes gain benefit for near and stationary distance vision tasks (e.g. blackboard and TV viewing) if a pinhole can be incorporated into the lens system.

Standard trial set pinholes are frequently of too small a diameter for this type of patient because of excessive light reduction. For trial purposes it is a simple matter to get a set of pinhole discs made in a range of diameters, e.g. 2, 4, 6, 8 mm. Initially one can try placing the pinhole disc in the back cell of a correctly centred trial frame, with and without trial lenses. This will indicate the effect of the pinhole on the visual axis with the eyes in the primary position. Many people cannot see through the pinhole in this position however and will need to hold the disc themselves. The potential value and optimal positioning of the pinhole can thus be ascertained.

A stenopaeic slit can sometimes be employed in a similar way (Fig. 3.1). Both pinholes and slits give an improved depth of focus and reduce scattered stray light. This may sometimes substantially improve acuity so that magnification can be reduced or occasionally dispensed with altogether.

(7)   *Varying light level effects on acuity*

Normal routine refraction examination is likely to have been conducted with comparatively low levels of ambient illumination, i.e.: with a semi-dilated pupil and no glare sources within the patient's visual field. Having recorded the VA under these conditions, increase the room lights and reposition the supplementary

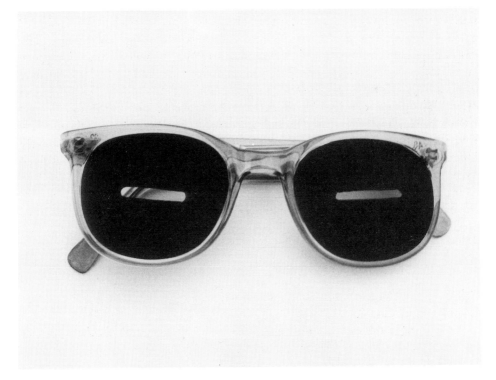

Fig. 3.1 Stenopaic slit spectacles.

lighting so that it becomes a glare source directed towards the patient's eyes. Record the VA again.

Most patients will find the glare source a bit unpleasant, but those with clear media or only peripheral opacities are likely to show unchanged or even slightly improved acuities with the bright light. On the other hand, the bright light-induced miosis may well result in a marked reduction in acuity in the case of patients with generalised media haze, central opacities or central field defects. Such people are likely to find their vision, and therefore their mobility, severely affected on bright sunny days and might well benefit from dark tinted spectacles, possibly with dark sideshields.

3.1.3   Alternative distance vision assessment charts

In the UK distance acuity is generally assessed by means of Snellen charts. These do have shortcomings when dealing with visually impaired people in that there is insufficient detail in the range commonly needed for such patients, i.e. approximately 4/60−6/36 acuity. The drawback is appreciably reduced if the chart is viewed at closer range − 3 m or 2 m distance. Alternative charts have been designed to minimise this problem. Unfortunately, few are readily available in this country.

(1)   Keeler A series distance card
        (Keeler, 1956)

Designed to be viewed at 3 m distance, it comprises non-serif letters based on a logarithmic scale such that each letter represents a constant fraction (80%) of the preceding letter. A vision grading of A2 represents 80% acuity compared to A1 acuity. Thus a patient with A2 acuity who wishes to see A1 detail requires magnification which will make A1 letters appear as large as A2 letters:

$$A2 = 1/0.8A1 = 1.25A1$$

Thus to raise acuity by one A unit requires 1.25 × magnification. To raise it by 'n' A units requires 1.25^n × magnification.

Table 3.1 Distance equivalents, Keeler A series compared to Snellen notation.

Keeler A unit @ 3 m	Snellen equivalent @ 6 m
A1	6/6
A4	6/12
A7	6/24
A11	6/60
A14	3/60

The 3 m distance card has 15 letter sizes, A1−A15, covering the more familiar Snellen range 6/6 to approximately 3/60. Thus there are two A letter gradings corresponding to the 3/60−6/60 Snellen range and three A sizes between 6/60 and 6/24 Snellen compared to the single intervening size (i.e. 6/36) actually available on a Snellen chart.

(2)   Sloan distance acuity chart
         (Sloan, 1959)

This American chart uses non-serif letters and has two acuity ratings between 20/100 (6/30) and 20/200 (6/60). It is designed for use at 20 feet but may be used at any desired closer distance.

The basic chart range comprises 13 steps from 20/200−20/13 (6/60− approximately 6/4) in approximately 0.1 log unit steps. Some letters are more easily recognised than others. Ten letters were selected, ZNHRVKDCOS, which have broadly similar levels of difficulty to each other and to a Landolt C ring, which is used as a reference standard.

(3)   Bailey−Lovie Chart Fig. 3.2
         (Bailey & Lovie, 1976)

This chart comprises 14 rows, each of five non-serif letters, ranging in size from 6/60 to 6/3 Snellen equivalent. It is designed to be viewed at 6 m range but converts easily to shortened viewing distances. It is a very logical chart. Adjacent lines differ in size by a factor of 1.26 (0.1 log unit). Spaces between letters are equal to the width of the letters on that line and the spaces between the lines equal the height of the letters in the smaller row, thus following the same logarithmic basis. The fact that each line incorporates five letters eliminates one of the other inconsistencies associated with conventional Snellen charts, namely that the top letter measures single letter acuity while the rest of the chart records linear acuity.

(4)   Waterloo Charts Fig. 3.3
         (Strong & Woo, 1985)

These charts are based on the Bailey−Lovie logarithmic principles but with a different letter layout. The person reads along the top line until a mistake is made, when the vision level is further investigated by reference to the vertical row of letters of the size causing difficulty.

There are five letters per row, and the chart is designed for use at 4 m distance. Letter selection from the basic Sloan optotypes has been made on the basis of ensuring equal interrow legibility. The black interaction bars round the

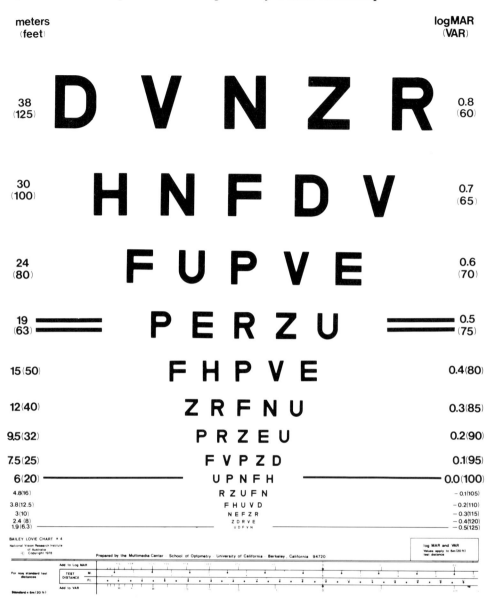

meters (feet)		logMAR (VAR)
38 (125)	**D V N Z R**	0.8 (60)
30 (100)	**H N F D V**	0.7 (65)
24 (80)	**F U P V E**	0.6 (70)
19 (63)	**P E R Z U**	0.5 (75)
15 (50)	**F H P V E**	0.4 (80)
12 (40)	**Z R F N U**	0.3 (85)
9.5 (32)	**P R Z E U**	0.2 (90)
7.5 (25)	**F V P Z D**	0.1 (95)
6 (20)	U P N F H	0.0 (100)
4.8 (16)	R Z U F N	− 0.1 (105)
3.8 (12.5)	F H U V D	− 0.2 (110)
3 (10)	N E F Z R	− 0.3 (115)
2.4 (8)	Z D R V E	− 0.4 (120)
1.9 (6.3)	U D F V N	− 0.5 (125)

BAILEY LOVIE CHART # 4
National Vision Research Institute of Australia © Copyright 1978
Prepared by the Multimedia Center   School of Optometry   University of California   Berkeley, California   94720

log MAR and VAR
Values apply to 6m (20 ft)
test distance

For non. standard test distances   TEST DISTANCE   M.   Fi.   Add to Log MAR   Add to VAR
Standard = 6m (20 ft)

Fig. 3.2   Bailey–Lovie distance vision chart. (*Courtesy of the authors and the NVRI, Australia.*)

edge of the chart are a further aid to standardisation. They ensure that the top and end-of-row letters are of equal difficulty to the rest of the chart in terms of single letter/linear acuity factors.

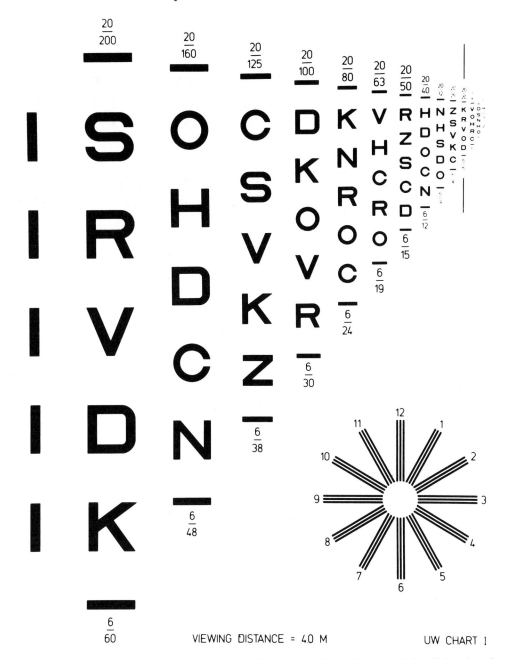

Fig. 3.3 Waterloo distance vision chart. (*Courtesy of the designers and the University of Waterloo, Ontario.*)

(5)   *Ferris–Logmar charts*
         (Ferris, Kassoff, Bresnick & Bailey, 1982)

This American chart, which was introduced in 1982, is based on Bailey–Lovie principles, utilising Sloan optotypes and recommendations of the Committee on Vision of the American National Academy of Sciences–National Research Council (1980). Ferris *et al.* (1982) who designed the chart have produced three versions, one for use during refraction, and one each for final VA measurement of R and L eyes. Basic design is for 4 m use, giving acuity gradings from 4/40– 4/2 (6/60–6/3) but it may be used at closer distances if necessary.

In Britain the Keeler A chart (supplier Keeler Ltd) is the most easily obtained alternative to the standard Snellen chart. None of the American charts is marketed in this country. Details may be obtained from the Lighthouse, Optical Aids Division, New York for the Sloan designs; from Berkeley, California and the University of Waterloo for Bailey–Lovie and Waterloo charts; and from Globe Screen Printing, Baltimore for the Ferris charts (Addresses: Appendix 5).

Visual acuity recording by means of the Snellen fraction is universally understood and accepted. Other systems encountered on occasion, in research work and in widespread clinical use elsewhere in Europe, are the decimal visual acuity and the logarithm of the minimal angle of resolution, LogMAR, and the minimal angle of resolution itself, MAR. Decimal visual acuity is obtained by dividing the numerator of the Snellen fraction by its denominator, i.e. 6/6 = 1.0; 6/12 = 0.5; 6/24 = 0.25; 6/60 = 0.1, etc.

The minimal angle of resolution for a given letter is obtained by inverting the Snellen fraction, i.e. a 6/24 letter subtends 1 minute arc at 24 m distance, if viewed at 6 m range it subtends 24/6 = 4 minutes arc. LogMAR is significant if using the American charts since they are based on 0.1 LogMAR differences between letter sizes and associated viewing distances.

(6)   *Low contrast visual assessment*

Research work in the last few years has produced considerable evidence of the value of low contrast visual assessment in the detection of a range of pathological conditions. The concepts involved are most easily understood by analogy with sound waves and radio channels.

Hearing assessment is carried out using sound of varying frequency. Impaired hearing may take the form of a loss of sensitivity to all frequencies, or a selective frequency range loss. A person might be unable to hear high pitched sound, for example, but respond reasonably normally to low frequency sound.

In a similar way, it is hypothesised that the visual system processes images by means of channels, 'tuned' to various types of visual stimuli (Blackemore & Campbell, 1969; Graham 1981). At retinal and visual pathway level the optical image giving rise to the visual stimulus is simply a geometrical pattern of edges of varying intensity light and dark zones.

For assessment purposes the stimulus is defined in terms of contrast and spatial frequency.

$$\text{Contrast (\%)} = \frac{\text{maximum luminance} - \text{minimum luminance}}{\text{maximum} + \text{minimum luminance}}$$

Contrast sensitivity (CS) is the reciprocal of the threshold contrast at which object/stripe can just be discriminated. Thus the lower the contrast, the higher the contrast sensitivity. Spatial frequency is the number of cycles (bright plus dark stripe) per degree visual angle subtense at the eye (Campbell & Maffie, 1974).

Conventional Snellen-based assessment provides a measure of only one aspect of visual function. It records the ability to respond to small detail and thus measures high contrast, high spatial frequency descrimination.

The ability to function in a general environment, to recognise faces, to move around, to perceive and to interpret large objects, is moderated by low frequency vision channels. Snellen VA measurements provide inadequate information about this aspect of the visual process.

Visual pathway dysfunction (including demyelinating disease, cortical lesions, glaucoma and amblyopia) can reduce the ability to see large objects while sparing small detail (Regan & Neima, 1983). A combination of CS and VA testing will obviously give a much more balanced assessment of overall visual function than is possible with conventional VA recording alone.

Stimuli used for CS assessment are either sine wave or square wave gratings or reduced contrast letters. Arden plates (Arden & Jacobson, 1978) marketed as the American Optical Contrast Sensitivity Test, and the Vistech Contrast Test System (Ginsburg, 1984) Marketed in the UK by Keeler, both use sine wave gratings. Cambridge Low Contrast Gratings (Wilkins, 1986) marketed by Clement Clarke International Ltd, use square wave gratings. Clement Clarke also manufacture the Pelli-Robson low contrast letter chart (Pelli, Robson & Wilkins, 1988).

Regan & Neima (1983) describe the use of low contrast letter charts, which they claim are as accurate as sophisticated sinewave gratings. Tunnacliffe (1989) outlines a similar chart found useful in routine optometric practice.

There is no doubt that CS assessment is potentially a very valuable diagnostic procedure. Further refinement, development and documentation of the actual tests is required, however, if the technique is to progress to become a routine part of optometric visual assessment (Reeves & Hill, 1987; Reeves, 1991).

When dealing with visually impaired patients, comparison of VA and CS findings can sometimes help to explain apparently contradictory findings. Most practitioners have experience of patients with acquired defects whose general visual abilities are much worse that would be predicted from consideration of VA and field measurement levels. Conversely, there are patients who function much better than expected, despite very low VA levels. The former group are likely to have much poorer CS discrimination abilities.

Faye (1986) feels that the pattern of response to low, medium and high spatial frequency ranges provides valuable additional data on visual performance. She suggests that CS, measured through alternative magnifiers, can be used to select the optimum unit.

Amber/yellow filters are sometimes beneficial in increasing contrast for patients suffering from macular degeneration or complaining of glare. CS measurements can give helpful objective information and guidance as to the best colour and intensity of any proposed tint.

CS can be a useful way of monitoring a disease process, but as Hess (1984, 1986) points out it has no differential diagnostic value in itself. He also considers that the use of large gratings is possibly misleading when the pathology is not even, and points out that the very controlled test conditions inevitably render it unrepresentative of real everyday conditions, e.g. with regard to light scatter.

Nevertheless, on balance, contrast sensitivity, even in its present underdeveloped state, is a helpful adjunct to a thorough visual assessment.

3.1.4   Establishing baseline near vision performance

Near acuity: reading acuity, alternative assessment systems.

(1)   Near acuity

The mathematical basis of the Snellen distance acuity system is that each letter subtends a 5′ arc visual angle when viewed from the specified distance.

Single letter near vision tests are available which record acuity in the same way, i.e. single capital letters viewed at a specified distance with letter size calculated to subtend multiples of the same 5′ visual angle unit.

A 'Reduced Snellen' chart is often included in British Faculty of Ophthalmology reading cards. The letter size is $\frac{1}{17}$th of its distance equivalent and should be viewed at 35 cm. The American Lighthouse near acuity test, which uses Sloan's M notation (see below), is also a single letter test system calibrated for 40 cm viewing distance.

Single letter tests measure the same thing regardless of the viewing distance involved. Thus, the distance and near acuity measured on this basis should be equal.

(2)   Reading acuity

Reading acuity is much more complex than near acuity. It requires a test based on complete words or continuous text, since it must measure the ability of the visual system to recognise groups of possibly blurred, distorted letters, and correctly to interpret them as words and sentences.

The earliest Jaeger near vision tests were non-standardised, with wide variation in letter and word spacing and type styles. This led to the widespread adoption of the Faculty of Ophthalmology approved reading tests (Law, 1952), based on the Times New Roman typeface. Size notation is based on the 'point' system of printing. One 'point' measures 0.353 mm or $\frac{1}{72}$ in. The measurement relates to the size of the carrier on which the letter is mounted. Actual size and angular subtense will vary with individual letters and print styles. Within any given print style there is a direct mathematical relationship between letter size notation, i.e. an N12 letter is half the size of an N24 letter, but there is no consistent size differential between adjacent sections of text on the testcard.

The major alternatives are the Keeler A system, designed for use at 25 cm distance, and the Sloan–Lighthouse, Bailey–Lovie and University of Waterloo charts, which all utilise a 40 cm viewing distance.

The *Keeler reading system* is based on the same logarithmic basis as the distance chart with each 'A' number representing a constant fraction of 80% of the acuity expressed by the preceeding number and magnification relating to the ratio of the letter sizes (Table 3.2).

Table 3.2 Magnification required to raise acuity when using Keeler 'A' series charts at 25 cm viewing distance:

Visual acuity	Magnification required to raise visual acuity to					
'A' series	A 10	A 9	A 8	A 7	A 6	A 5
A6						1.3
A7					1.3	1.6
A8				1.3	1.6	2.0
A9			1.3	1.6	2.0	2.5
A10		1.3	1.6	2.0	2.5	3
A11	1.3	1.6	2.0	2.5	3	4
A12	1.6	2.0	2.5	3	4	5
A13	2.0	2.5	3	4	5	6
A14	2.5	3	4	5	6	8
A15	3	4	5	6	8	10
A16	4	5	6	8	10	12
A17	5	6	8	10	12	15
A18	6	8	10	12	15	18
A19	8	10	12	15	18	23
A20	10	12	15	18	23	

From Keeler Manual: *Helping the Partially Sighted*.

The *Sloan–Lighthouse* system comprises five cards with text in graded sizes from 1M to 5M. 1M lower-case letters subtend 5′ arc visual angle at 1 m distance, 10 M subtend 5′ arc at 10 m distance and so on. 1 M print approximates to N8 in actual size, but when viewed from the specific viewing distance of 40 cm is equivalent to distance acuity of 6/15. This in turn equates to vision necessary to resolve N5 print at 25 cm range.

The Bailey–Lovie word card (Fig. 3.4) uses the printing 'point' N system and Times New Roman type style, but selects print size on the same logarithmic basis as is used for their distance chart. Print sizes range from 2 point (i.e. N2) up to 80 point (N80) in 15 stages. When viewed at the standard distance of 40 cm this equates to 6/3.8–6/150 distance acuity, or 6/6–6/240 distance acuity if the word card is read at 25 cm distance (see Table 3.3). The card also has a logMAR conversion scale which is read directly if viewed from 25 cm range.

Each card measures 26 cm × 20.6 cm and contains the full range of print sizes in one block of disconnected words, i.e. not continuous text. A selection of 20 cards is available to prevent patients memorising the words!

The University of Waterloo near vision test card (Fig. 3.5) almost manages to combine all permutations for near assessment on to one card! There is a continuous text reading section, four normal contrast letter or symbol panels and two low contrast letter panels all based on Bailey–Lovie/LogMAR size and

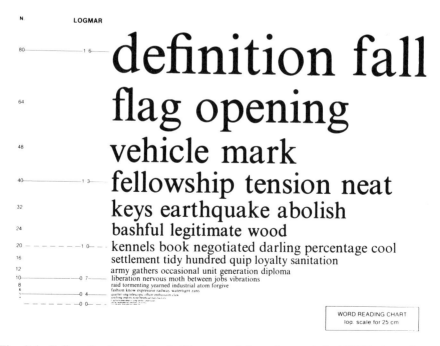

Fig. 3.4 Bailey–Lovie word card. (*Courtesy of the authors and the NVRI, Australia.*)

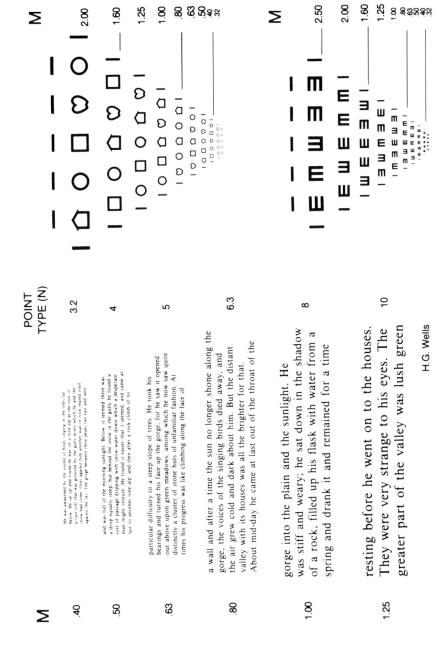

Fig. 3.5 University of Waterloo near vision test card. (*Courtesy of the designers and the University of Waterloo, Ontario.*)

spacing principles. The continuous text section is of marginal value in work with low vision patients since it is confined to small print sizes. Table 3.3 provides a comparison of the various alternative assessment schemes available.

Whichever system is employed for near vision assessment it will generally be found that normally sighted people record distance, near and reading acuities which correlate well with each other.

As may be seen from Table 3.3, for optometrists using the N series charts held at approximately 25 cm, there is a very useful 'rule of thumb' which provides a helpful mental starting point when turning one's attention to a patient's near vision requirements. The denominator of the corrected Snellen distance VA, if divided by 3, will give a good approximation to the equivalent N-near vision standard one would expect to achieve with the appropriate reading addition. Thus 6/36 = N12; 6/24 = N8; 6/18 = N6.

In the case of visually impaired people the nature of the ocular problem will affect the visual performance such that the reading acuity is frequently inferior to the single letter near acuity, and theoretical predictions often collapse in

Table 3.3 Comparison of alternative near acuity assessment systems related to their equivalent distance acuity values.

		Equivalent visual acuity scales			
Distance vision notation		Near vision notation			
Snellen fraction		Times New Roman and Bailey–Lovie N or 'point' unit		Keeler A Series	Sloan Lighthouse M units
American	English				
		at 25 cm	at 40 cm	at 25 cm	at 40 cm
20/10	6/3		2 pt		
20/20	6/6		3 pt	A1	
20/25	6/7.5		4 pt	A2	M0.5
20/30	6/9		5 pt	A3	
20/40	6/12		6 pt	A4	
20/50	6/15	N5	8 pt	A5	M1
20/60	6/18	N6	10 pt	A6	
20/80	6/24	N8	12 pt	A7	
20/100	6/30	N10	16 pt	A8	M2
20/120	6/36	N12	20 pt	A9	M2.4
		N14		A10	
20/160	6/48	N18	24 pt	A11	M3
20/200	6/60		32 pt	A12	M4
20/240	5/60	N24	40 pt	A13	M5
20/300	4/60	N36	48 pt	A14	M6
20/400	3/60	N48	64 pt		M8
20/600	2/60		80 pt	A17	M10

practice! Macular problems for example can give rise to disproportionate reading difficulty in comparison with the distance VA. Theoretical mathematical relationships are useful nonetheless; an adult patient achieving a significantly better than expected near acuity should lead one to recheck the distance refraction!

3.1.5   Recording near vision performance

Near vision measurements should be carried out with a good, even illumination on the test card. Consideration and demonstration of the effects of improved task illumination will be a vital part of the instruction to the patient, but at this stage the light levels should not be boosted excessively. To do so would give an unrealistic, inflated near VA baseline value atypical of the patient's normal visual performance. Acuity should be recorded monocularly and binocularly.

In the absence of sufficient accommodation the appropriate working distance addition must be provided. One can use a trial frame or lenses in a Halberg clip over existing distance spectacles as appropriate. Single vision lenses are to be preferred where possible rather than bifocals, owing to the latters inevitably restricted reading area.

The accommodation/addition is obviously 2.50D if the Sloan 40 cm charts are being used and 4.00D for 25 cm range vision. Times New Roman N charts can be held at either distance depending on the practitioner's preference. Calculations and comparisons associated with magnification requirements do however tend to be less complicated if the shorter distance is adopted (see Chapter 5).

Knowledge of the acuity and the visual requirements enable the optometrist to predict the magnification likely to be required for various tasks.

3.1.6   Supplementary near tests

(1)   Amsler chart

The Amsler grid is a valuable way of deriving a picture of the function of the macular and paramacular areas. Viewed at 30 cm with near correction, it covers the 10° field surrounding fixation, i.e. the central 20° of the visual field. The information regarding scotomas is useful in its own right but in LVA work we are often more interested in locating the areas of least distortion, i.e. the least damaged sections of central retina capable of the clearest vision. This is essential information if the eccentric viewing techniques described in Chapter 7 are to be employed in the visual retraining of the patient.

(2)   Colour vision assessment

It should be remembered that within the population as a whole, approximately 8% of males have some degree of inherited red−green colour vision defect.

Colour discrimination declines with age as a normal adjunct to crystalline lens sclerosis. The most marked loss of sensitivity is at the short (violet−blue) wavelength end of the spectrum.

Detailed colour vision assessment is of course undertaken for diagnostic purposes and to monitor the progress of a retinal or neurological disease process. In the context of a LVA assessment colour vision testing should be attempted for children (especially boys) whenever practical.

Realistically, however, it is not usually very informative in the case of elderly patients with acquired vision defects. It tends merely to confirm the existence of a problem that you knew to be inevitable in view of the site of the lesion and the age of the patient.

Advice and suggestions to minimise the problems caused by defective colour discrimination will be of benefit to the great majority of visually impaired patients. It is a particular problem for diabetic patients who rely on colour vision for their daily urine tests to monitor their diabetic control. A comprehensive discussion of the investigation, occupational and educational implications, and management of colour problems may be found in 'Defective Colour Vision' (Fletcher & Voke, 1985).

Armed with the refractive details, distance and near acuity, visual field and general supplementary information and the detailed picture of the patient and his or her major problems, the practitioner is in a position to embark on the actual selection and assessment of optical aids in the first place, followed by advice and suggestions of a more general nature to assist the person make the best use of their residual vision.

3.2   Assessment routine for children

3.2.1   Babies and pre-school age groups

Assessment is obviously very limited in comparison to that of an adult, but two visits may nevertheless be required. Young children have a very short attention span and a very low boredom threshold. It may well be advantageous to carry out whatever general investigative procedures and unaided vision measurements are possible at the initial visit, but to defer cycloplegic refraction, ophthalmoscopy and VA (where feasible) to a separate occasion. Two visits are preferable to risking the head-on confrontation with a bored, tired toddler which can result from an overly protracted examination session.

A paediatric ophthalmologist may order electrodiagnostic tests or an ocular/fundus examination under anaesthetic for a child about whom there is serious concern. Within an optometric consulting room context investigations and measurements will be dictated largely by the age and comprehension of the child.

(1)   History

Parents, and experienced health visitors, may suspect a problem from the child's behaviour and development. This is by no means always the case however. I know of two multi-handicapped little girls with the same general medical syndrome. The parents could not be persuaded to bring the younger child for assessment until she was nearly two years old, despite her elder sister having had bilateral cataracts diagnosed and operated upon by the age of 6 months. The parents were convinced that the younger child could see normally and were devastated to be told that she also had dense bilateral cataracts.

Birth details, any abnormalities or infections during pregnancy, general medical problems and any known family ocular problems, are all highly relevant whenever a visual defect is suspected in a child.

(2)   General appearance and pupil reflexes

- Any obvious facial asymmetry?
- Any obvious squint?
- Are the pupil reflexes normal?
- Does the child show any interest in the unfamiliar surroundings?

It may be obvious that the child is looking around and taking an interest in what is going on round it. The pen torch used for pupil reflexes should elicit a response. If not what happens if the room is darkened, the angle-poise light moved around and directed towards the child's eyes? Does the child object to the very bright light – a normal reaction – or does it provoke a positive response in the case of a child who had 'ignored' the pen torch and other less visually stimulating objects? This reaction would lead one to suspect one was dealing with a child with a fairly significant visual problem. The final alternative is that the very strong light produces no reaction, which points towards a massive visual deficit.

(3)   Cover test and oculomotor status

A Hirschberg (corneal reflex) test may be all that is possible, although near cover tests with a light or interesting toy can be attempted. One's hand or thumb is usually the best occluder! Motility by means of a light or squeaky toy or brightly coloured glove puppet, etc., should be attempted. There is likely to be a significant amount of head movement but it should still be possible to detect any gross restriction of ocular movement.

Fusional movements, and thus the development of binocular function, can be checked by interposing base out prism before each eye in turn. The suggested range is 10^Δ for up to one year old and 20^Δ at age two to three years (Edwards,

1988). Failure to elicit a response to such tests again suggests the existence of impaired visual function and development.

(4)   Vision assessment

Alternate occlusion: observing the child's response when each eye is covered in turn for a short while will give a good indication of any major difference in vision between the two eyes. Observation of the child's general reaction to the environment, to lights, coloured toys, Smarties, and so on, all give a guide to the visual status.

Catford Drum: moving dots or stripes of varying sizes elicit an optokinetic response if resolved by the visual system. The test will give an indication of acuity from a few weeks of age upwards. Some authorities however feel it overestimates the acuity by a factor of 4 for emmetropes and possibly even more for myopes (Atkinson *et al.*, 1981).

Preferential looking techniques: encouraging results have been obtained in clinical trials for a number of years (Atkinson *et al.*, 1982) although standardised consulting room tests have become available only recently.

The American Teller Acuity Cards and the Keeler Acuity Card Assessment Set (Fig. 3.6) both utilise contrast sensitivity style grating targets calibrated in cycles/degree and Snellen equivalents.

There are obvious problems with a young baby's attention span, but the technique is reputed to give reliable results between two and nine months of age. Beyond nine months of age, on the whole, normal children are simply too wriggly for any meaningful results! Visually impaired children, or others with delayed development may sometimes respond to the test at an older age (Fig. 3.7).

Stycar ball test: for slightly older babies, 6–9 months of age. White polystyrene balls are either rolled across the floor or held out on the end of a rod from behind a screen. The observer watches for a response from the child to the appearance of the balls which are reduced in size until no response is elicited or the child gets bored and 'opts-out'.

Matching tests: picture matching tests are appropriate for children from around two years of age. Kay (1983) single symbol and Elliott (1985) linear picture tests are constructed on Snellen optotype principles and as such are a significant improvement on the earlier Beale–Collins type pictures. Such tests are generally performed at 3 m distance.

Picture tests lead on to Sheridan–Gardiner single letter, Ffooks symbols,

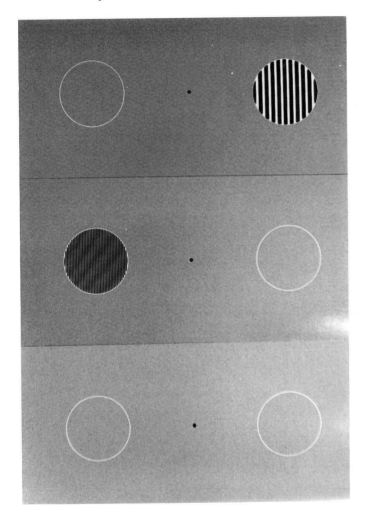

Fig. 3.6 Examples from the preferential looking, Keeler Acuity Card Assessment set. Grating targets approximately equal to Snellen acuity 6/250 (20/800), 6/60 (20/200), 6/18 (20/60). (*Courtesy Keeler Ltd.*)

Landolt-C and Illiterate E tests. These tests come into the same general category of matching tests but have the added complication of requiring a reasonable degree of manual dexterity on the part of the child.

(5) Cycloplegic refraction

Small degrees of astigmatism and comparatively modest amounts of hypermetropia (approximately 2D) are encountered routinely in normal small children. Cyclo-

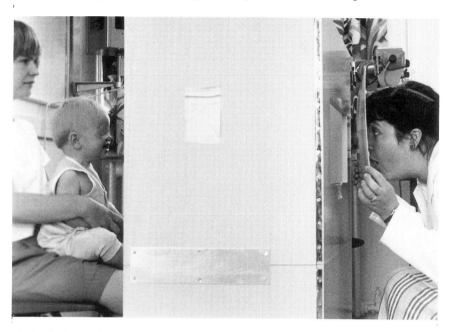

Fig. 3.7 Keeler preferential looking test in use. The observer watches the child through the small hole in the centre of the test card as it is placed in position. Target contrast is reduced until there is no discernible response from the child. (*Orthoptic Clinic, Coventry & Warwickshire Hospital.*)

plegic examination is essential to obtain any degree of accuracy. Premature and very tiny babies may exhibit high, variable amounts of myopia and marked astigmatism which resolves within the first few months of life. Beyond this stage, anisometropia in excess of 1.00D and markedly atypical levels of refractive error warrant more careful monitoring. Spectacle correction may well be necessary to minimise the possibility of the child developing refractive amblyopia. If the child is old enough to tolerate a trial frame, corrected VA measurements can be attempted.

(6)   *Ophthalmoscopy*

It is sensible to take advantage of the pupil mydriasis at this stage of the examination. In normally fixing children one tends to get an excellent view of the macula and little else! Indirect ophthalmoscopy often gives a more extensive, though still very fleeting glimpse of the fundus than is possible with a conventional direct ophthalmoscope.

The age guidelines associated with various vision tests relate to normally sighted children of average intelligence. Under normal circumstances a child receives the overwhelming majority of its information about the world around it through its eyes. Psychological and intellectual development, motor skills and co-ordination all rely in large measure on visually received stimuli. To a greater or lesser extent a visually impaired child is deprived of this visual stimulation. All aspects of its development are liable to be retarded. This in turn renders accurate visual assessment even more difficult than normal.

In addition it is now recognised that some children suffer maturational delay of the visual system or cortical processes (Hoyt *et al.*, 1983).

Occasionally, children may be encountered in whom no visual function can be demonstrated in the first months after birth but normal vision develops thereafter.

The difficulties of accurately assessing and predicting long term visual abilities mean that most ophthalmologists are very reluctant formally to register a young child blind or even partially sighted. It is vitally important nevertheless that visual problems are detected early. Parents can then hopefully be put in touch with social workers, home teachers, RNIB specialists and so on, to receive support and advice on creating a visual environment to provide maximum visual stimulation and potential for development for the child.

3.2.2   Refractive correction of partially sighted children

Significant refractive errors should be corrected from an early stage to encourage maximum development of the visual pathways.

It should be remembered however, that a partially sighted child with active accommodation has the potential for a vastly superior near vision performance in comparison to an elderly person with a similar pathology and similar distance acuity. The child will instinctively hold objects close to the eyes and utilise accommodation to focus the retinal image. Thus they function with a built-in magnifier. 10D accommodation equates to 2.5 × magnification in standard terminology.

Children generally also have clear media. Light levels reaching the retina are correspondingly higher so illumination is not likely to be such a critical factor in their near vision performance. Children may have distance acuities within the partially-sighted (and sometimes even full blind) categories, yet have near acuities at very close range that are only a little below normal.

The exception to this general observation is any child with defective accommodation of congenital or surgical origin or secondary to systemic disease or medication. Aphakic children for example will have a near vision potential which is very similar to the equivalent aphakic adult.

Such children should be given bifocal spectacles as soon as possible. The segment should be fitted higher than normal to enhance near vision performance, with a reading add power generally at least +4.00D. This enables the child to hold objects comparatively close and to benefit from the resulting larger retinal image size. It also takes account of the sometimes overlooked fact, that small children have short arms!

Prior to this stage it is arguably better to give an aphakic baby or young child a single vision, overpowered close range prescription in preference to a distance prescription. Infants and young children have a comparatively close range environment. Visual stimulation comes predominantly from near objects. Development of visual acuity, hand-eye co-ordination and other motor skills, interest in toys, etc., is likely to be encouraged by refractive correction appropriate to the approximately 20−75 cm range involved. It is most important that parents understand what is being done. They can then ensure that as far as possible the child is physically in the centre of activity, to inject the maximum visual stimulation and information into its environment.

3.2.3   Assessment of older children

Assessment accuracy improves immeasurably as soon as linear Sheridan−Gardiner tests can be carried out reliably. More exact cover-tests and oculo-motor evaluation become feasible and Frisby and Titmus stereopsis tests can be considered for those with only mild visual impairment.

Colour vision assessment should be attempted as soon as possible. Much infant and junior school teaching is colour coded. It is clearly important that parents and teachers be aware of any particular colour vision anomaly affecting the child.

A general point should be made about examination of children with nystagmus. Nystagmus is present in a high percentage of children with congenital ocular disorders. It is essential to record binocular VA for both distance and near vision, with the child allowed to adopt whatever head position they instinctively prefer. Binocular VA is frequently superior to the monocular VA of either eye, and there may be considerable variation with head position. The child who consistently adopts a very extreme 'abnormal head posture' to minimise the amplitude of the nystagmoid movement should be referred for ophthalmological opinion with a view to extra-ocular muscle surgery.

Amplitude of the nystagmus reduces when the eyes converge (Abadi & Sandikcioglu, 1975). Near acuity may therefore be a little better than expected in comparison with distance acuity. On the other hand, amplitude increases with tension, stress or ill-health, so a nystagmus patient's performance can vary considerably depending on the circumstances in which they find themselves.

3.3   Summary

It may be seen that the refractive examination of a visually impaired child or adult evolves naturally from the refractive routine applied to a normally sighted individual. Most adaptations are common sense – the use of larger lens power 'steps', higher power cross-cycls, charts at closer distances and a more deliberate, slower approach and so on. The aim is the same after all, regardless of the level of vision, namely to establish the optimum refractive correction. For a normally sighted patient this culminates in recommendations regarding spectacles. Our visually impaired patient may also benefit from spectacles, but the refractive result, plus information from supplementary tests (pinholes, Amsler grid, etc.) forms the foundation for the more specific optical low vision aid assessment.

The refractive findings must be allied to knowledge of the patient's problems and requirements, established in the course of the expanded 'history and symptoms' questioning.

Technical information regarding the availability, scope, and limitations of optical aids is integrated with the composite 'picture' of the patient. One will then hopefully be in a position to conduct a productive assessment, of maximum benefit to the patient, both in terms of optical help and general advice.

Questions

1   In what ways would you expand the normal 'history and symptoms' questioning when dealing with a visually impaired person?
(See Section [3.1.1].)

2   What analogy might you use to explain to a patient:

(a) a media problem?
(b) a retinal problem?

(See Section [3.1.1] (5).)

3   What modification might you make to your normal ret/subjective refractive routine to accommodate the needs of a patient with poor sight?
(See Section [3.1.2].)

4   What do you know about alternatives to the standard Snellen acuity charts? Are there alternatives to the Times New Roman N near charts?
(See Sections [3.1.3] and [3.1.4].)

5   What is the 'rule of thumb' for relating distance and near acuity?
(See Section [3.1.4] (2).)

6   Which supplementary tests might profitably be included in the assessment routine?
(See Section [3.1.2] (6); [3.1.2] (7); [3.1.6] (1); [3.1.6] (2).)

 7 How would you assess a visually impaired pre-school child?
   (See Section [3.2].)

 8 In what way does the near vision potential of a child differ from that of an elderly person with a similar ocular problem?
   (See Section [3.2.2].)

 9 What policy would you adopt towards the refractive correction of aphakic toddlers?
   (See Section [3.2.2].)

10 Why is it particularly important to establish binocular acuities in the case of a patient with nystagmus?
   (See Section [3.2.3].)

CHAPTER 4

Distance Vision: Magnification and Management

It is generally impractical to provide distance vision magnification with a single lens, although hypermetropic patients will gain some magnification effect if spectacles are supplied with a large vertex distance. However, distance vision magnification normally requires a telescopic lens system. In LVA work we use either the Galilean or modified astronomical telescope systems.

4.1 Galilean telescope system

4.1.1 Basic design

This system comprises a positive objective lens and a negative eyepiece lens separated by the difference between their focal lengths (Fig. 4.1).

When intended for LVA use, this design has the advantages of producing an upright image in a small, compact, lightweight unit. This is balanced by the disadvantage of low magnification and a comparatively restricted field of view.

4.1.2 Magnification considerations

$$\text{Magnification of telescope} = \frac{-F_e}{F_o} = \frac{-f_o}{f_e}$$

It is therefore possible to obtain a specified magnification with many differing pairs of lens powers, bearing in mind that the tube length (i.e. the size of the unit) is also directly related to the lens powers used.

Example: Galilean telescope 2× magnification

(1) F_o +1.00DS
    F_e −2.00DS   Unit length 50 cm

(2) F_o +10.00DS
    F_e −20.00DS   Unit length 5 cm

(3) F_o +20.00DS
    F_e −40.00DS   Unit length 2.5 cm

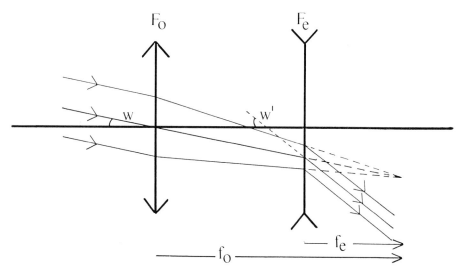

Fig. 4.1 Ray diagram – Galilean telescope.
Objective lens: dioptric power F_o focal length f_o
Eyepiece lens: dioptric power F_e focal length f_e
Angular magnification $= \frac{W'}{W}$

Use as an LVA requires a compact system necessitating high powered lenses. This in turn introduces significant spherical and chromatic aberrational problems and poses practical limits to the lens diameters which can be used. These factors result in a practical limit of approximately $3\times$ magnification for an afocal distance Galilean telescope intended for LVA use. At greater magnification levels than this the image quality, field and light gathering properties are so poor that the unit is unlikely to be of much use.

If on the other hand the telescope were designed to be stand mounted, with no restriction on its physical size, high magnifications would be quite feasible. For example F_o +1.00DS, F_e −10.00DS gives $10\times$ magnification with a tube length of 90 cm. Hardly a practical proposition for an LVA!

4.2 Astronomical telescope

These are also known as Keplerian telescopes.

4.2.1 Basic design

A positive objective lens combined with a positive eyepiece lens separated by the sum of their focal lengths. Fig. 4.2.

The basic telescope unit produces a magnified real image. Unfortunately, it is

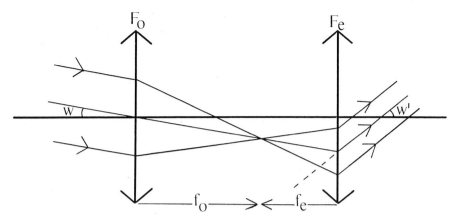

Fig. 4.2 Ray diagram – Astronomical telescope.
Objective lens: dioptric power F_o focal length f_o
Eyepiece lens: dioptric power F_e focal length f_e
Angular magnification $= \frac{W'}{W}$

inverted (i.e. upside down) and reversed (right for left). It is necessary to incorporate an additional lens or prism system to 're-invert' and 're-reverse' the image. The frequent use of some form of correcting prism gives rise to the description often applied to this type of unit as a 'prismatic' or 'roof prism' binocular or monocular telescope.

When compared with the Galilean design, an astronomical telescope for LVA use has the advantage of greater magnification and improved image quality with a proportionately greater field of view. The disadvantages concern the greater size and weight; inevitable consequences of the greater separation between objective and eyepiece lens, and the need for the supplementary lens or prism system.

4.2.2 Magnification considerations

Available in $4\times$ to $10\times$ magnification range in monocular or minaturised binocular form. The most frequently used options are $6\times$ and $8\times$. The lower lens powers enable slightly larger diameter lenses to be used and lens aberrations are less severe. Thus light gathering properties and image quality in an astronomical system are generally superior to those of a Galilean telescope.

4.3 Optical considerations in telescope design

The clinical low vision aid practitioner does not need to become excessively involved in complex optical considerations of telescope design. However, awareness of some of the basic principles of apertures, stops and pupils is helpful in understanding how such factors affect

(1) The ability of the system to transmit light and
(2) the field of view.

4.3.1 General definitions

Aperture stop or *entrance pupil*: opening in the optical system which effectively limits the amount of light flux from an axial point which can enter the system. In a telescope/eye system this will usually be the objective lens.

Field stop: opening in the optical system which effectively limits the field of view. Usually the eyepiece lens.

Exit pupil: image of the aperture stop as formed by the eyepiece lens.

4.3.2 Image brightness

In the case of both systems the aperture stop is the objective lens and the field stop is the eyepiece lens. The relationship between the diameters of these two lenses affects the light gathering properties of the telescope.
    The optimum situation arises when the diameters are in the ratio:

$$\frac{\text{diameter of objective lens}}{\text{diameter of eyepiece lens}} = \frac{f_o}{f_e} = \text{magnification of unit}$$

    Providing the ratio is maintained, the larger the lenses, the greater will be the amount of light transmitted through the system and the brighter the axial image. Increasing the diameter of either lens without a corresponding increase in the size of the other will not improve image brightness.
    Many telescopes utilise anti-reflection coated lenses to maximise light transmission and image brightness.

4.3.3 Field of view

The size and position of the exit pupil determines the theoretical field of view of a telescope. In practical use the telescope/eye system is a little more complex. The key to the actual performance of the unit is the position and size of the exit pupil relative to the entrance pupil of the eye. For telescope alone:

$$\text{diameter of exit pupil} = \frac{\text{diameter of objective lens}}{\text{magnification of unit}}$$

Knowledge of the lens powers and position and separation within the unit enables the exit pupil position to be calculated or established by ray tracing methods (Fig. 4.3 and Fig. 4.4).
    The manufacturer's specification of the field of view of a telescope is a

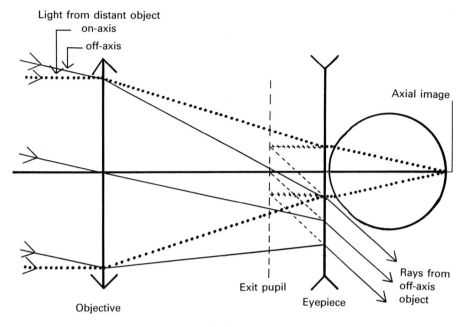

Fig. 4.3 Exit pupil and field of view: Galilean telescope.

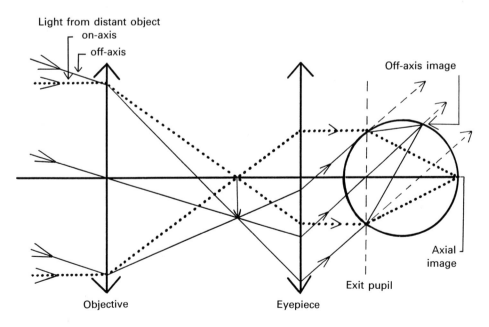

Fig. 4.4 Exit pupil and field of view: Astronomical telescope.

theoretical, mathematical calculation. It is technically correct but does not represent the realistic performance for the telescope in use.

The Galilean system negative eyepiece gives rise to a virtual exit pupil within the optical system (Fig. 4.3). The astronomical system produces a real exit pupil in space beyond the eyepiece lens (Fig. 4.4). Maximum field of view is achieved when the exit pupil of the telescope and the entrance pupil of the eye are coincident. In addition, all light entering the aperture stop/entrance pupil leaves the system at the exit pupil. An eye positioned at that point will benefit from maximum light intensity and image brightness.

A coincident exit pupil and eye is readily attained with an astronomical telescope but is clearly an impossibility with the Galilean design. The manufacturer's specification is likely to be a reasonable guide to the practical field of view in use in the case of the astronomical telescope. A Galilean unit, on the other hand, will have an actual performance which is very much inferior to that suggested by the theoretical calculations (Table 4.1).

Fig. 4.5 is an example of the limited field of view inherent in the high power, small aperture, miniaturised distance telescopic systems used in low vision aid work.

The telescope field of view is further reduced if the user wears spectacles. As may be seen from Table 4.1, the effect is relatively small in the case of units of Galilean design. Since the exit pupil is invariably considerably in front of the user's eye, moving the telescope forward to fit over a spectacle lens does not produce too marked a reduction in the field of view.

Moving an astronomical unit 10−15 mm away from the eye to accommodate spectacles, however, wrecks the exit pupil/eye pupil relationship and severely reduces the field.

The diameter of the exit pupil should ideally be a little larger than the diameter of the ocular pupils, so that the pencil of rays from the telescope slightly overlaps the eye's pupil. Unfortunately, the constraints of the comparatively small lens apertures and high powers required to construct a compact unit for LVA use, results in a small exit pupil diameter (2.5 mm in 4 × 10 and 8 × 20 units, up to 3.75 mm in 8 × 30 unit).

A small exit pupil renders telescope alignment quite critical. Slight hand shake or telescope movement will result in the emergent light pencil missing the eye pupil. The object would then vanish. The greater the disparity between eye and exit pupil position, the more acute the problem. It is thus a significant problem for spectacle wearers, who are trying not to scratch glasses and having to contend with a smaller field of view as well!

These different exit pupil positional effects are easily visualised and understood by simply considering the field of view and ease of alignment when holding a pinhole disc close to one's eyes compared to an inch or so away.

Table 4.1 Field of view measurements in a selection of hand-held or spectacle-clip mounted distance telescopes. A comparison of manufacturer's technical specifications with actual measured values obtained with units in use by (i) emmetropic and (ii) spectacle wearing, observers. Vision/VA 6/5. Results illustrate the marked field reduction experienced by spectacle wearers when using astronomical telescopes, due to moving the exit pupil plane further away from the plane of the eye pupil. The practical field of view was found to be less than the theoretical level for almost all units tested.

Unit Specification	Manufacturer's details		Measured values Unaided		Measured values In spectacle plane	
	Field of view (degrees)	Linear field at 100 m distance	Field of view (degrees)	Linear field at 100 m distance	Field of view (degrees)	Linear field at 100 m distance
Keeler multicap Ref51 distance unit 1.75×			18½°	33½ m	16½°	30 m
Keeler Clip, Ref 40 2×, Galilean focusing			9°	16 m	8½°	14½ m
Eschenbach 3 × 23 Ref. 4492 Galilean	9°	16 m	7°	12½ m	7°	12½ m
Roof prism monoculars						
4 × 12	12.5°	22 m	11°	20 m	7°	12½ m
6 × 16	10°	17½ m	9°	16 m	4½°	7½
8 × 20	6.5°	11½ m	7°	12½ m	3½°	6 m
10 × 30	6°	10½ m	6°	10½ m	2½°	4½ m
Miniature binoculars						
Viking 8 × 20 ZWCF	8.2°	14½ m	7°	12½ m	5½°	9½ m
Viking 6 × 15 micro	7°	12½ m	6½°	11½ m	6°	10½ m

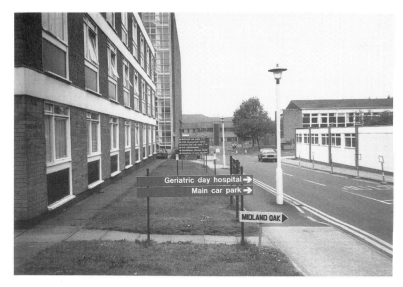

(a)

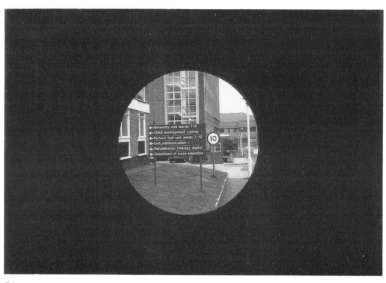

(b)

Fig. 4.5 Illustration of the field of view obtained with distance vision telescopic units. Direction board and surroundings, as seen by a normally sighted person, compared with the reduced field of view and magnified image obtained from the same viewpoint when using a 2× Galilean and 4× and 8× Astronomical design monoculars. This also illustrates the significantly better field of view characteristics of Astronomical compared to Galilean telescope optical design. (a) Field of view − normally sighted observer. (b) 2 × 23 monocular Galilean telescope design. F of V 9°. (c) 4 × 12 monocular Astronomical telescope design. F of V 11°. (d) 8 × 20 monocular Astronomical telescope design. F of V 7°.

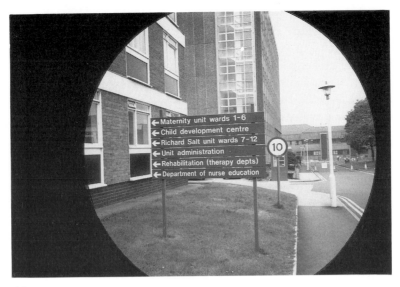

(c)

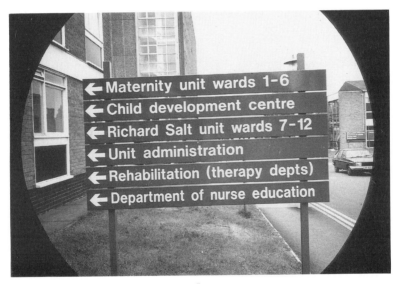

(d)

4.4 Principles of variable focus systems

Many units have a small amount of eyepiece focussing adjustment to enable the user to compensate for his own (spherical) ametropia. As discussed earlier, the field of view will be enhanced if there is sufficient adjustment to enable the person to use the telescope without spectacles since the eye's pupil and the exit pupil will be more nearly coincident.

Where a high level of ametropia and/or astigmatism renders this impossible, the spectacle prescription may sometimes be incorporated into the eyepiece lens. However, it is often impractical to keep removing spectacles when using the telescope. One tends to run out of hands!

The basic distance telescope is an afocal system. It receives parallel incident light and produces a parallel emergent beam. If, however, the telescope is directed towards a comparatively near object, the divergence of the incident light is magnified through the system to give a very divergent emergent light beam. An eye trying to see even intermediate range objects with a distance telescope would require substantial accommodation to focus this divergent light. Dowie (1988) gives a useful empirical 'rule of thumb' for Galilean telescopes designed as LVAs (i.e. with short tube length and high powered lenses).

Such units give rise to the approximate relationship:

$$\text{Accommodation required (D)} = (\text{magnification of unit})^2 \times \text{dioptric equivalent of viewing distance}$$

e.g. $2\times$ Galilean telescope, viewing object at 25 cm distance

$$\text{Accommodation required} = (2)^2 \times 4 = 16\text{D}.$$

Thus standard distance telescopes really are distance vision aids only. On the other hand there are many occasions when the user is interested in rather nearer objects — notice boards, road names, signposts, etc. — in the intermediate, 3 feet–10 feet (90 cm–3 m) viewing range. This requires modification of the basic afocal distance optical system to overcome the problem of the divergent emergent light.

The necessary modification may be achieved in one of two ways. A very high powered plus lens could be interposed between the telescope eyepiece and the user's eye. This is theoretically reasonable, but practically foolish, because of the well-known problems of aberration, reduced lens apertures and poorer image quality associated with high powered lenses.

A much more sensible option is to place a plus lens over the telescope objective lens. This supplementary lens will be of low power since it is only necessary to neutralise the divergence of the light incident on the telescope objective. Rendering it parallel re-establishes the basic afocal optics. The additional power may be provided by a lens cap, giving clear vision at specific distances fixed by the power of the cap, or by varying the objective – eyepiece separation.

The extremely useful variable focus option is achieved by a design which incorporates an adjustable tube length in order to produce the different lens separations. As the tube length (i.e. the lens separation) increases, the objective lens power effectivity becomes greater, giving clear object focus at steadily closer range.

Such units are usually known as focussing or extra-short focus telescopes and have a range from infinity to approximately 25 cm.

4.5 Range of distance telescopic units available

4.5.1 Fixed-focus systems (Fig. 4.6)

There is a small range of compact Galilean spectacle mounted units such as the Rayner Telecap units, Bier-Hamblin and Zeiss telescopic spectacles and the Keeler multi-cap telescope. They are restricted to a modest magnification in the order of 1.75× to 2×.

More powerful units are astronomical/Keplerian optical systems. Currently,

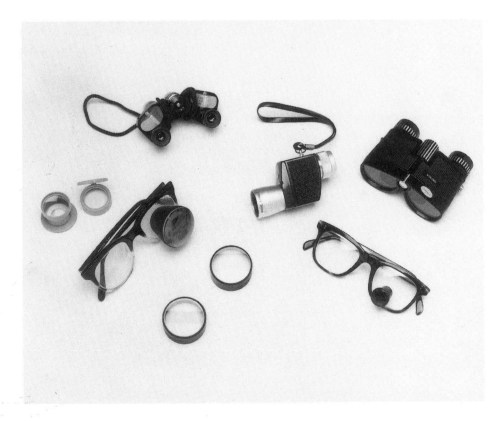

Fig. 4.6 Fixed focus distance monocular and binocular telescope units. Hand held: 6 × 15 binocular; 8 × 24 miniscope; 8 × 20 ZWCF binocular (available from Viking Optical Ltd; Edward Marcus Ltd). Spectacle mounted: Keeler Multicap; Rayner Telecap; and Zeiss 2× magnifying spectacles.

the Zeiss 3.8× telescopes are spectacle mounted but all other units are more bulky and are intended for hand-held use. Magnification of 6× and 8× is available in monocular or miniaturised binocular form.

4.5.2   Variable focus telescopes (Fig. 4.7)

There is a rather greater choice of focussing telescopes, with the range including monocular and binocular spectacle mounted aids as well as the hand-held versions and monocular units with finger-ring or spectacle clip mountings.

Miniature 2× Galilean systems are available hand-held (with finger-ring) or spectacle mounted with focussing range, ∞ to approximately 40 cm. Eschenbach produce a 3 × 23 Galilean telescope, (range ∞ to 70 cm) binocular form in a lightweight adjustable-PD frame or as a monocular unit in a spectacle clip for spectacle wearers. Keeler supplement their Galilean based units with three

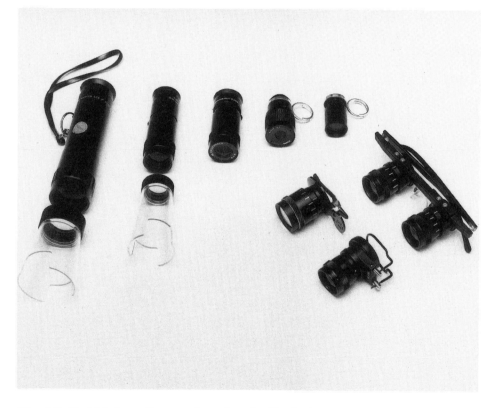

Fig. 4.7   Variable focus distance telescopic units. Roof prism monocular units, 10 × 20 and 8 × 20, shown with microscope attachment; 6 × 16 unit; (Viking Optical Ltd; Edward Marcus Ltd); Keeler 4.2 × 12; 2× finger ring and 2× Clip telescope; Eschenbach 3× clip or binocular spectacle unit (Associated Optical).

panfocal telescope-monoculars. The 2.8× (range ∞ to 16 cm) and 4.2× (range ∞ to 30 cm) are spectacle mounted or hand-held. The much larger 8.25× unit (range ∞ to 30 cm) is hand-held only.

Some larger monoculars are produced with a conventional hard plastic casing or optionally with a thicker, softer 'rubber-armour' coating which provides much greater protection in the event of the telescope being banged or dropped.

Most importers and suppliers feature a range of extra-short focus roof-prism monoculars. The lettering on the casing may vary but the technical specification of the various ranges are identical (Table 4.2).

Table 4.2 Roof prism, extra short focus monoculars.

Unit spec	Focus range infinity to:	Mounting					
		Finger ring	Spectacle clip	Spectacle mounted	Hand held	Microscope attachment	Rubber armour
2.75 × 8	15 cm	√	√	√			
4 × 10	20 cm	√	√				
4 × 12	20 cm	√	√	√		√	
6 × 16	26 cm	√	√	√	√	√	
7 × 25	50 cm				√		
8 × 20	30 cm				√	√	√
8 × 30	60 cm				√	√	√
10 × 20	40 cm				√	√	
10 × 30	70 cm				√	√	√

4.6   Patient assessment

The comparatively limited range of appliances simplifies assessment. Nevertheless there are several factors to take into account when helping the patient select the most appropriate telescope for their needs:

(1)   Basic distance acuity.
(2)   Sizes and distances of objects of interest.
(3)   Monocular *v.* binocular considerations.
(4)   Manual dexterity and steadiness.
(5)   Cost.

Points (1) and (2) determine the magnification required. It may be necessary to spend a little time establishing what the particular problem areas are and what the person needs, or would like to be able to see. (Not always the same thing!)

The range of viewing distances will determine the need for a fixed or variable focus unit.

An adult with a mixture of visual requirements is likely to need a variable short-focus unit. A younger child, whose prime need is seeing the blackboard, may actually find a variable focus unit too complicated. Such children are often much better with a fixed-focus unit which cannot be 'fiddled-with'.

Point (3): monocular *v.* binocular units: a monocular unit is generally satisfactory when patients have a significant difference between the acuities of their two eyes. Those with more symmetrical defects and a full field, e.g. albinism and nystagmus, may prefer a binocular unit. Binocular viewing gives an improved field of view and may stabilise nystagmus and improve VA. Binocular units may also be of value for people with patchy field defects such as occur in cases of diabetic retinopathy. Binocular vision may enable the brain to employ the jigsaw principle, superimposing the two imperfect images to enhance the resultant visual quality.

If considering a monocular, it is advisable to assess acuity with the unit using each eye in turn. Usually, but not invariably, the person elects to use the eye with the better basic acuity. Occasionally this is not the case. The relative position and sizes of field defects, allied to magnification can sometimes give unexpected results. Patients may also have a preference for using the dominant eye even if it actually has the poorer acuity.

The first task after all is to locate the object of interest in the field of view of the telescope. Ocular dominance and 'handedness' certainly can play a part in the ease with which a person can 'get their bearings' when viewing through a telescope.

Point (4): a steady hand and reasonable manual dexterity is an essential prerequisite to successful use of a hand-held unit. Those with shaky hands may well have to sacrifice magnification in order to use a spectacle mounted unit.

Point (5) cost: units are loaned to patients through the Hospital Eye Service. Individual departments may be subject to budgetary restraints and for a non-health service patient cost may well be a factor that has to be taken into account. In general:

- Binocular units are more expensive than monocular units.
- Variable focus designs are more expensive than fixed-focus units.

4.7   Patient training

A fortunate few patients will have the benefit of advice and help from a mobility officer who can incorporate use of a telescope into their own individually designed mobility training programmes. Sadly the majority of patients are handed a telescope and left to cope on their own.

Whatever type of telescope is used the patient needs help to master efficient focussing, scanning and tracking techniques. Any normally sighted person who has used a conventional pair of binoculars knows how frustrating it can be, trying to locate the object of interest. This already tricky task becomes far more difficult if someone is contending with poor vision and field defects in addition to the restricted field of the telescope.

Interdisciplinary programmes in Europe and America, and the results achieved recently in Britain by the training programmes of the Partially Sighted Society, demonstrate clearly that a patient's best interests are served if a broadly based functional assessment is combined with a training programme in the use of the aids supplied. (Backman & Inde, 1979; Collins, 1987)

Telescopic units normally are never worn while walking around. Spectacle or head-mounted units are used while seated or for stationary tasks. Hand-held devices are used as spotting aids. For example, the person, having arrived at the station, gets the monocular out to check the departure boards or timetable (Fig. 4.8).

Handling and manipulation, particularly of variable focus units, need to be

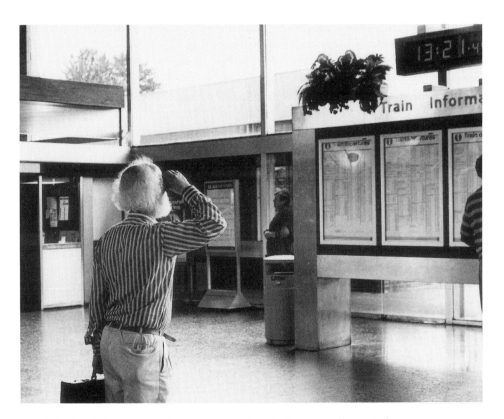

Fig. 4.8 8 × 20 monocular in use as a spotting device at a railway station.

practised. It is important to acquire the knack of adjusting the focus and using the telescope with one hand. If both hands have to be used the person has constantly to stop and put down shopping, handbag, briefcase, etc., before being able to use the telescope. Clearly this is undesirable. It slows down activity considerably and belongings are inclined to get overlooked and left behind, trodden on by other pedestrians, or stolen, while the owner's attention is elsewhere. With practise it is possible to use one finger to gauge the width of the groove in the telescope casing and learn to relate this to the corresponding focussing range. Since the user knows the approximate distance of the object of interest, the telescope focus can be almost 'pre-set' manually in advance, leaving only the fine adjustment to be done while actually looking through the unit. This significantly speeds up reaction times and improves general efficiency of performance.

Once basic manipulative skills are understood, advice and training in logical, systematic scanning and tracking techniques should begin. Initially, indoors people must learn to discipline themselves to scan the environment using steady horizontal sweeps until the object of interest is located. Experience and common sense usually determine the starting point. If an object is generally on the lower part of a wall, start at floor level and work up. Adopt the opposite procedure for items which experience suggests are usually higher up — start scanning at the roof or ceiling and work down. The person must use the brain to help the eyes. Randomly waving the telescope around in the general direction of the object is useless!

With forethought and practise it is possible to learn to locate moving objects such as bus numbers. The user focusses the telescope on a fixed object — a building, a window, a road sign or whatever is convenient — which is at the approximate height of the number on the bus. This fixed object should be as far away as possible to give sufficient reaction time. Once the telescope has been focussed on this object, periodic sweeps are made across the road at this level until the bus appears. Smooth adjustment of the telescope then enables the number to be kept in focus for long enough for it to be read accurately and appropriate action to be taken (Fig. 4.9).

This level of expertise will only be acquired with patience and practice. The initial instruction and training is in itself time-consuming and people may need a great deal of encouragement and support before they acquire the confidence to go out and travel independently.

It is not normally a practical proposition for optometrists engaged in LVA work to become involved with a patient to this extent. Ideally, there should be established lines of communication with local mobility officers so that they are informed of any patient issued with a telescope for the first time, or indeed of any patient who would seem to be in need of mobility training.

Unfortunately, mobility officers are in very short supply. In many areas of the

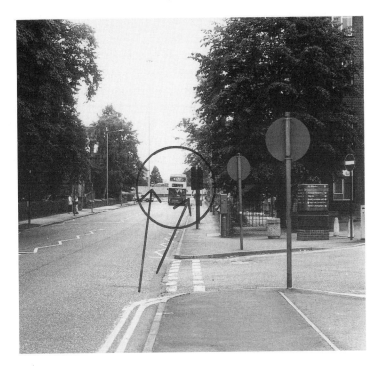

Fig. 4.9 While waiting for the bus, the person lines up the distance telescope on a suitable fixed object, e.g. no-entry sign or the edge of traffic lights. As the bus approaches, the number/destination board will 'put itself' into the field of view of the telescope, giving the person time to take appropriate action.

country no satisfactory service exists. Where this is the case, advice and limited practical help from the LVA clinic optometrist is infinitely better than no help at all.

4.8   Summary

The practitioner's role is:

(1)   To establish the patient's needs and advise on units that are available.
(2)   To explain, compare and contrast units.
(3)   To make it clear to the patient what is possible and what is optically impossible. Everyone wants a high-powered, compact unit with a large field of view!

A sense of reality must, however, be maintained. Sadly there are many elderly people with acquired visual defects who are incapable of using a telescope because of their general mental or physical infirmity. Independent mobility outdoors would not be a practical possibility for them even if they had normal sight. For such people telescopes are simply not appropriate.

Where they may be of benefit, the practitioner must allow the patient to try the various units so that the relative merits can be assessed in each individual case. The final decision must rest with the patient. As much advice and training as possible must then be offered to enable the person to gain the maximum benefit from the telescope.

Follow-up appointments must also be arranged to allow the aid selection to be confirmed, or for reassessment, if necessary, based on the person's experience of actually using the aid.

Questions

1. Explain the basic optical principles of the Galilean and astronomical telescope systems.
    (See sections [4.1] and [4.2].)

2. How much magnification can be offered for LVA use with these two alternative systems?
    (See section [4.5].)

3. What factors influence the field of view of a telescope?
    (See section [4.3.3.].)

4. How may a distance telescope be modified for intermediate or near use?
    (See section [4.4].)

5. What factors might influence your recommendations concerning monocular or binocular units?
    (See section [4.6].)

6. What sort of instruction would you give a patient concerning use of the telescope?
    (See section [4.7].)

CHAPTER 5

Near Vision: Mathematical Considerations – Hand and Stand Magnifiers

5.1 Mathematical aspects of near vision magnification

5.1.1 Definitions

For any given object there are three different ways in which magnification may be achieved (Fig. 5.1).

(a) Relative size magnification: increase the size of the object by non-optical means.
(b) Relative distance magnification: move the object closer to the eye.
(c) Angular magnification: increase the visual angle subtended by the object at the eye by optical means.

Linear magnification

However the magnification effects are achieved, the linear magnification is the ratio of image size to object size.

Definition of magnification is a complicated and much disputed topic. It is possible to become involved in detailed calculations concerning object: image position, size, available accommodation, lens form and so on (Bailey, 1980, 1981; Bennett, 1977, 1982). Such calculations are, of course, theoretically valid and of considerable interest to those with a mathematical turn of mind. In reality, such technical minutiae have little relevance to day-to-day LVA practice. Clinicians should be familiar with concepts of magnification rating and classification as they apply to the units they use. This involves understanding the basic nominal magnification formula and its relationship to the test distance used (see section [5.1.2]) and the newer idea of maximum magnification (see section [5.1.3]). Any suggestion of a need for more mathematical expertise should be 'debunked'.

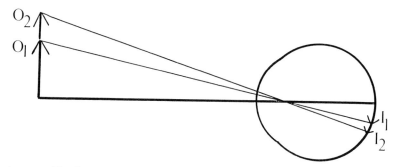

(a)   Relative size magnification.

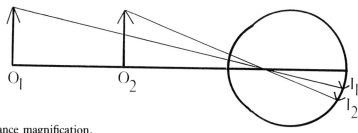

(b)   Relative distance magnification.

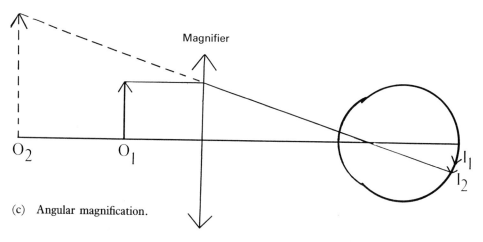

(c)   Angular magnification.

Fig. 5.1 Diagrammatic representation of alternative methods of achieving near vision magnification. O_1 is the initial reference size and position of an object which gives rise to a retinal image, size I_1. O_2 is the new size or position of the object which gives rise to an enlarged retinal image, I_2.

5.1.2   Nominal magnification

This is also sometimes referred to as 'effective magnification' or 'conventional magnification'. To avoid unnecessary complexity at this stage, thin lens theory will be assumed.

This form of angular magnification is based on the widely used concept of 'least distance of distinct vision', i.e. a standard distance at which it is assumed a suitably corrected normal eye could comfortably view print. Most manufacturers and most texts about magnification base their work around a 'least distance of distinct vision' of 25 cm.

The patient is assumed to have any distance refractive error corrected and to have a reading addition or accommodation to focus an object clearly at 25 cm distance (i.e. a total near addition of +4.00D). Since the retinal image size is proportional to the angle subtended at the eye by the object, the retinal image size under these conditions is taken as the reference against which the retinal image size from the magnified object is to be compared. These standardised conditions are said to have unit magnification, i.e. magnification = 1.

Thus the use of the standard 25 cm notional distance gives rise to the conventional nominal magnification formula:

$$\text{Nominal magnification of a lens} = \frac{F}{4}$$

where F is the dioptric power of the lens

It should be stressed that this use of a 25 cm 'least distance of distinct vision' *is* only an arbitrary convention. Some practitioners feel that a longer working distance is more realistic and prefer to base their work and calculations on a working distance of 33 cm or 40 cm (Sloan−Lighthouse system). One can make out a very reasonable case on clinical grounds for the longer working distances. Most normally sighted individuals adopt a reading distance of between 30−40 cm, comparatively few would choose to hold a book as close as 25 cm naturally. It has to be recognised however, that lens manufacturers do use the 25 cm, $\frac{F}{4}$, system as the basis for their calculations. Use of a longer 'least distance of distinct vision' working distance has the inevitable practical disadvantage that the practitioner must recalculate the magnification rating of all instruments and units used.

$$\text{Working distance 33 cm: nominal magnification} = \frac{F}{4}$$

$$\text{Working distance 40 cm: nominal magnification} = \frac{F}{2.5}$$

The mathematical theory of the nominal magnification formula is given below for information.

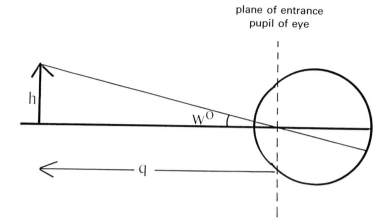

(a) Object h, at 'least distance of distinct vision' q, angular subtense at eye, w°.

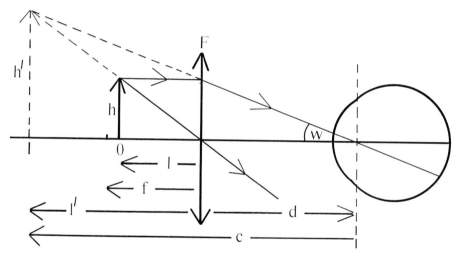

(b) Object h, placed with the anterior focal point of lens F, gives rise to an upright, magnified, virtual image h', angular subtense at eye, w.

Fig. 5.2 Nominal magnification.

Theory: nominal magnification

Linear magnification: $\dfrac{h'}{h} = \dfrac{-l'}{-l} = \dfrac{L}{L'}$

Ref. Fig. 5.2 $\tan w° = \dfrac{h}{-q}$ and $\tan w = \dfrac{h'}{(-l' + d)}$

$$\text{Angular magnification } M = \frac{\tan w}{\tan w°}$$

$$M = \frac{h'}{(-l' + d)} \div \frac{h}{-q}$$

$$= \frac{h'}{4h} \times \frac{-q}{(-l' + d)}$$

$$= \frac{L}{L'} \times \frac{-q}{\left(-\dfrac{1}{L'} + d\right)}$$

$$= \frac{qL}{1 - dL'}$$

Special case: an object placed at the anterior focal point of lens will give rise to an image at infinity.

$$\text{i.e. from Fig. 5.2 } -1 = -f; \ L = F;$$
$$l' = \infty; \ L' = 0;$$

$$\text{Thus angular magnification } M = \frac{qL}{1 - dL'} = -qF$$

$$\text{e.g. } q = -25\,\text{cm} = -\frac{1}{4}\,\text{m} \quad M = -\left(-\frac{1}{4}\right) F = \frac{F}{4}$$

$$q = -40\,\text{cm} = -\frac{1}{2.5}\,\text{m} \quad M = -\left(-\frac{1}{2.5}\right) F = \frac{F}{2.5}$$

5.1.3   Maximum magnification

This is also referred to as iso-accommodative magnification (Bennett, 1977, 1982) or manufacturer's magnification.

   This is a definition based on the premise that the hand or stand lens is positioned and used in such a way that the object–lens–eye system produces an image at the least distance of distinct vision, again taken to be 25 cm.

From Fig. 5.3, (a) and (b), it may be seen that:

$$\text{Angular magnification } M = \frac{\tan w}{\tan w°} = \frac{qL}{1 - dL'}$$

$$\text{when } -q = (-l' + d)$$

$$M = \frac{(l' - d)\,(L' - F)}{1 - dL'}$$

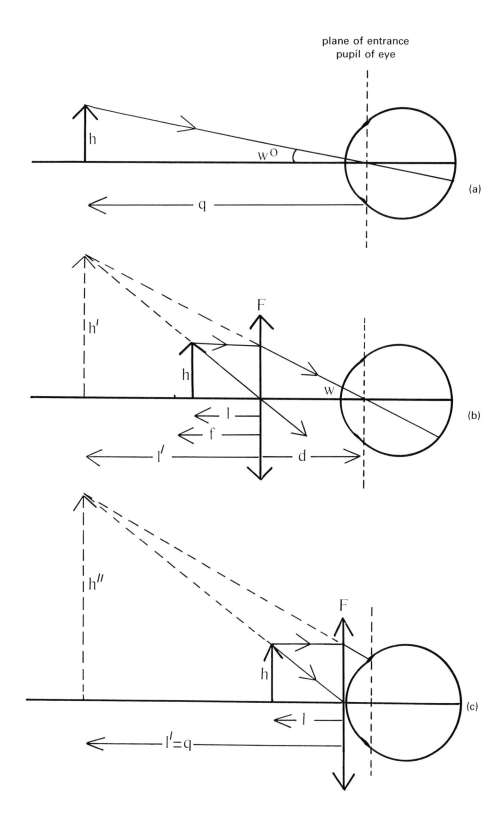

plane of entrance
pupil of eye

w^o

h

q

(a)

F

h'

h

w

l

f

l'

d

(b)

F

h''

h

l

l' = q

(c)

$$= \frac{(1 - dL') - (l'F - dF)}{1 - dL'}$$

$$= 1 - \frac{(l'F - dF)}{(1 - dL')}$$

$$= 1 - l'F$$

$$= 1 - (q + d) F$$

Maximum magnification (Fig. 5.3(c)) is achieved under the theoretical condition that the magnifying lens F is in contact with the eye.

$$M = 1 - (q + d) F$$

When d = 0, $M = 1 - (q)F$

if q = 25 cm, $M = 1 + \frac{F}{4}$

An easier, although mathematically incorrect way of thinking about maximum magnification is:

A lens, power F, positioned so that it gives rise to an image 25 cm away from the eye.
+ the eye requires 4.00D accommodation/spectacle addition to focus the image.
= the combined system: comprising the nominal magnification of the lens $\left(\dfrac{F}{4}\right)$

plus the accommodation/reading add power magnification effect $\left(\text{i.e: } \dfrac{4}{4} = 1\right)$,

giving a maximum magnification of $\dfrac{F}{4} + 1$.

Increasingly manufacturers have adopted this maximum magnification rating for their lenses.

These two basic equations, $\dfrac{F}{4}$ and $\dfrac{F}{4} + 1$, are an adequate guide for clinical comparative purposes. However, both are only exactly true under conditions which do not normally occur in reality. Namely, that the object is held at the principal focus of the lens and that the magnifier itself is in contact with the eye to give a zero lens–eye separation!

The reality is of course that the object is always held within the principal focus and the lens is always a finite distance from the eye. Thus no two people using the same magnifier will experience the same magnification effect.

Fig. 5.3 (*opposite*) Maximum magnification. (a) Object h at least distance of distinct vision q. (b) General case: image h′ formed by lens F at distance q from eye. (c) Special case: image h″ formed at distance q from eye when lens F in contact with eye.

5.1.4   Dioptric power measurement and lens form

Another major complication arises because of the absence of any universally accepted convention for specifying something as fundamental as the basic lens power. Power can be recorded in terms of back vertex power (BVP), front vertex power (FVP) or equivalent power (F_e). For low power thin lenses the differences are negligible. Unfortunately, magnifiers are high powered, thick, highly curved lenses, so the differences are quite significant. Manufacturers' literature blandly states 'magnification or 'power' without elaboration, and it is not clear which of the three alternative power measurements is being used (Fig. 5.4).

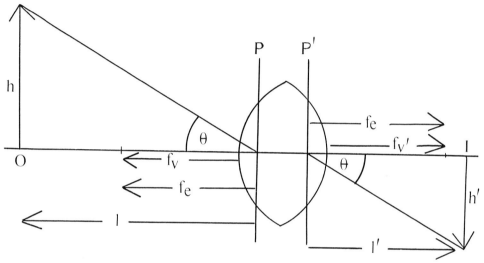

Fig. 5.4 Vertex power and equivalent power.
P − primary principal plane; P′ − secondary principal plane;
f_v − front vertex focal length; f'_v − back vertex focal length;
f_e − equivalent focal length.
Object O, size h, distance 1 from P subtends angle θ at P.
Image I, size h′, distance 1′ from P′ subtends angle θ at P′.
If 1 is large, such that O may be assumed to be at infinity, then $1' = f_e$.

Front and back vertex powers can be measured directly on a focimeter (providing the magnifier will physically fit onto the instrument) or may be established by neutralisation or calculation.

$$F_v = F_1 + \frac{F_2}{1 - \frac{d}{n'}\,F_2} \qquad F'_v = F_2 + \frac{F_1}{1 - \frac{d}{n'}\,F_1}$$

Where F_v = Front vertex power (DS)
         F'_v = Back vertex power (DS)

F_1 = Front surface lens power (DS)
F_2 = Back surface lens power (DS)
d = Lens thickness (m)
n' = Refractive index of lens

The equivalent power is the dioptric distance between each principal plane and the corresponding focal plane of the system.

$$F_e = F_1 + F_2 - \frac{d}{n'}\, F_1\, F_2$$

In the case of an equiconvex lens, FVP = BVP, but neither equals F_e. In the particular instance of a plano-convex lens F_e approximates closely to the FVP. For all other forms of thick lens, FVP and BVP differ from each other and from F_e. F_e is the same regardless of direction (i.e. there is no front and back F_e). Unlike FVP or BVP, F_e provides a precise indicator of lens performance since it relates directly to the angular size of the image. The angle subtended by the object at the front principal plane is equal to the angle subtended by the image at the second principal plane. With the exception of plano-convex lenses, it is not possible to measure F_e directly on a focimeter. However, Bailey (1981) describes an optical bench system for determining F_e which is applicable to single plus lenses, compound lenses or telescopic units. An object of known size, a known distance from the lens unit gives rise to an image whose size and position is measured. In the special case of parallel incident light the image will be formed in the equivalent focal plane of the unit. In practical terms the object distance is being measured to the front surface of the magnifying unit, not to the first principal plane, and the object is not at optical infinity. However, providing the object distance is large compared to the focal length of the test unit, the errors introduced are insignificant.

Rumney (1989) describes a nice consulting room adaptation of Bailey's ideas. An illuminated test chart forms the object (of known size and distance), whose image is formed directly on a ruler. Object and image sizes, and object distance once established, enable image distance to be calculated. The large object distance having been equated to parallel light, enables the image distance to be equated to f_e. F_e of the test unit is then the reciprocal of f_e (in metres) (Fig. 5.5).

If manufacturers were to adopt equivalent power for all magnifier measurements it would clarify matters considerably. If nominal magnification were invariably $\dfrac{F_e}{4}$ we would all know what was going on!

As the system stands at present, manufacturers may choose to rate lenses in terms of FVP, BVP or F_e, such that two units described as having the same magnifying power, may in fact be of significantly different dioptric power. This will obviously give rise to different amounts of angular magnification and often

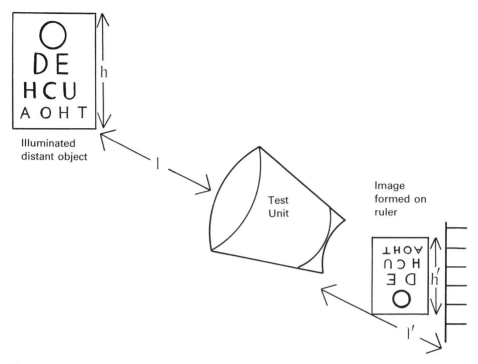

Fig. 5.5 Consulting room method of establishing F_e of a single or compound lens, or telescopic unit. The test chart, an illuminated, distant object (size h, object distance 1) is focussed by the unknown lens/unit to form an image directly on a ruler (size h′, distance 1′ from test unit). If 1 is large compared to 1′, then 1′ may be equated directly with f_e. Thus $F_e = \frac{1}{f_e}$ (in metres) (Rumney, 1989).

accounts for the very marked dissimilarity which frequently exists between supposedly equal strength units.

Lens form also varies. Bi-convex, plano-convex or aspheric single vision lenses, aplanatic and achromatic doublets and triplets are all represented within the magnifier ranges available. There are many different approaches to designing aspheric surfaces, depending on the relative importance attached to minimising spherical aberration or the oblique aberrations such as oblique astigmatism and distortion. This all adds further variability to the overall performance of the various commercially available lenses.

Lens materials also vary. Plastics, possibly with a scratch resistant coating, is the most commonly used material. Crown glass and regular glass (which has a characteristic green tinge) are used for some units, particularly high powered, small aperture lenses.

5.1.5   Object − lens separation effects

The greatest magnification occurs, as has been established, if the object is held at, or in reality fractionally within, the first principal focus of the lens giving rise to emergent light which is effectively parallel. In this situation the person should use distance spectacles and must maintain a non-accommodative state despite the near nature of the stimulus. Unfortunately, this greatest magnification is associated with the minimum field of view and the maximum disturbance from peripheral aberrations; chromatic aberration and pincushion distortion being particularly troublesome.

As the object is moved progressively closer to the lens the magnification decreases and the emergent light becomes steadily more divergent. It becomes necessary for the patient to accommodate or use reading glasses to overcome this divergence. The reduced magnification is associated with an improved field of view and less intrusive aberrational effects.

Most stand magnifiers are manufactured so that the stand height is less than the principal focal length of the lens. A child accommodates to overcome the resultant divergent light. A presbyopic person should use a stand magnifier with reading glasses. Variation between manufacturers with regard to the stand height selected for similar power lenses adds to the uncertainty, such that the manufacturer's quoted magnification rating bears only a token resemblance to the actual magnification achieved in use.

5.1.6   Lens-eye position and field of view (Fig. 5.6)

In an eye-magnifier system the pupil of the eye is the field stop. Hand or stand magnifiers are generally held at a 'normal' reading distance of approximately 25−35 cm. At this distance even quite large aperture lenses subtend a comparatively small angular subtense at the eye, e.g. a 100 mm diameter lens viewed at 30 cm has an angular subtense of about 18° (approximately $32^\triangle$). As a result, for most magnifiers used in this way, rays from across the whole aperture of the lens enter the pupil of the eye. Peripheral rays are subject to significant amounts of aberration despite the possible use of aspheric surfaces. This effectively reduces the field of view through the lens, giving a clear central area surrounded by a badly distorted peripheral zone.

Assuming the object − lens distance is kept constant, the closer the eye approaches to the lens the better will be the field of view. A magnifier much closer to the eye subtends a much larger angle and the pupil then acts as a pinhole, scanning across the lens aperture. This improves image quality and effective field by cutting out peripheral aberrational effects.

As we have seen, patients often prefer to hold objects well inside the principal

(a) ESCHENBACH 4x, 6x, 8x, Stand units.

Eschenbach 2627 4× lens
Ø 60 mm, F = 12D
Stand height: 45 mm to
underside of lens.
Field of view:
29 mm @ 15 cm viewing distance
26 mm @ 25 cm viewing distance
22 mm @ 40 cm viewing distance

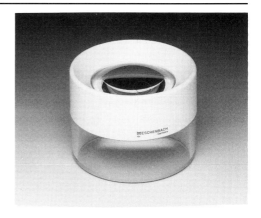

Eschenbach 2626 6× lens
Ø 50 mm, F = 20D
Stand height: 35 mm to
underside of lens.
Field of view:
24 mm @ 15 cm viewing distance
20 mm @ 25 cm viewing distance
18 mm @ 40 cm viewing distance

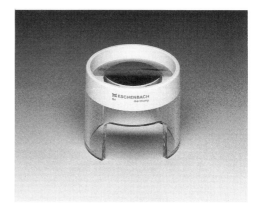

Eschenbach 2624 8× lens
Ø 35 mm, F = 28D
Stand height: 30 mm to
underside of lens.
Field of view:
13 mm @ 15 cm viewing distance
11 mm @ 25 cm viewing distance
8 mm @ 40 cm viewing distance

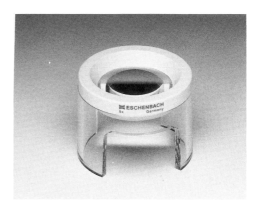

Fig. 5.6 (a) Illustrated F of V of Eschenbach 4×, 6× and 8× magnifiers with photographs and technical details of lenses concerned.

uce an image only about six times poorer than our own ∢

A EYES

of all vertebrates follow a similar design, which can be
camera. In land animals, the transparent window at the
cts like the ⸱t of a camera lens and bends or refra
This refract $4 \times$ because light travels at a different sp
lowever, ⸱ light is roughly the same in the co
; cornea simply protect the eye without bending the ligh
l the cornea is a pigmented area known as the iris, wh
he rays pass through a hole in the iris, called the pupil, ⸱
cally to alter the amount of light entering the eye, just a
djusts its aperture. Behind the iris is the curved lens, and th
ier air or water. The lens projects the light onto the retir
age. Fish bring the image into focus in a similar way to
towards or away from the retina. Mammals adjust the
is bulge me ⸱ning it.
cused light $6 \times$ ⸱ic of rod- or cone-shaped light d
tina. Each r⸱ contains a photo-sensitive pigmen
es when exposed to light cause a signal to be passed to n
tina. The retinal nerve cells process some of the informa
the optic nerve to the brain. For example, the human eye
cones, and the retina codes and combines the data so t
llion fibres entering the optic nerve.
rain not or ⸱ image the right way up, but als
of detail. $8 \times$ this, only one word at a time is
receive a ⸱ ⸱n of our surroundings, and can
field of view. The brain is so good at filling in, that altho
of our image is blurred and lacks detail and colour, we ⸱
yes of primitive vertebrates do much more of the pro
ypes of retinal nerve cells, each sensitive to different comp

Fig. 5.6 Experimental determination of the field of view obtained through a selection of fixed stand magnifiers. Emmetropic young observer, VA 6/5, viewing angle normal to the plane of the lens. Field of view determined for three pairs of equally rated magnifiers, eye-lens distances 15 cm, 25 cm, 40 cm. Field of view shown actual size.
Eye-lens distance: 15 cm — — — — — — — —
　　　　　　　25 cm _____
　　　　　　　40 cm . . . .

(b) COIL 4x, 6x, 8x, Stand units.

COIL 5214 4× lens
Ø 80 mm, F = 12D
Stand height: 77 mm to
underside of lens.
Field of view:
52 mm @ 15 cm viewing distance
35 mm @ 25 cm viewing distance
28 mm @ 40 cm viewing distance

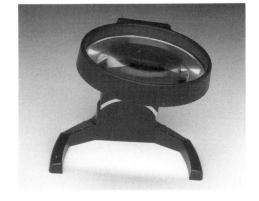

COIL 4206 6× lens
Ø 50 mm, F = 20D
Stand height: 43 mm to
underside of lens.
Field of view:
20 mm @ 15 cm viewing distance
14 mm @ 25 cm viewing distance
10 mm @ 40 cm viewing distance

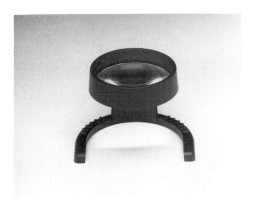

COIL 4208 8× lens
Ø 44 mm, F = 28D
Stand height: 33 mm to
underside of lens.
Field of view:
12 mm @ 15 cm viewing distance
8 mm @ 25 cm viewing distance
5 mm @ 40 cm viewing distance

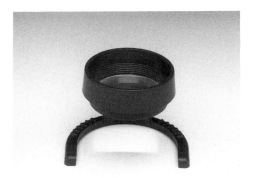

Fig. 5.6 (b) Shows similar data for COIL 4×, 6× and 8× magnifiers.

luce an image only about six times poorer than our own

.A EYES

; of all ver   low a similar design, which can be
camera. In **4x** als, the transparent window at the
.cts like the   at of a camera lens and bends or refr:
This refraction occurs because light travels at a different s[
However, the speed of light is roughly the same in the cc
s cornea simply protects the eye without bending the ligl
d the cornea is a pigmented area known as the iris, wl
The rays pass through a hole in the iris, called the pupil, v
ically to alter the amount of light entering the eye, just a
idjusts its aperture. Behind the iris is the curved lens, and th
her air or water. The lens projects the light onto the retir
nage. Fish bring the image into focus in a similar way to
towards or away from the retina. Mammals adjust the
ns bulge more, or flattening it.

ocused light l   c of rod- or cone-shaped light d
etina. Each ro **6x** ontains a photo-sensitive pigmen
es when expc   t cause a signal to be passed to n
etina. The retinal nerve cells process some of the informa
the optic nerve to the brain. For example, the human eye
l cones, and the retina codes and combines the data so t
illion fibres entering the optic nerve.

brain not only   1age the right way up, but als
of detail. As y **8x** s, only one word at a time is
receive a clear   of your surroundings, and can
field of view. The brain is so good at filling in, that altho
: of our image is blurred and lacks detail and colour, we (
eyes of primitive vertebrates do much more of the pro
:ypes of retinal nerve cells, each sensitive to different comp

focus, sacrificing magnification in the interests of a better field of view. If, however, this alternative means of improving field is adopted, i.e. holding the lens much closer to the eye, it will be found that the object can be moved back, nearer to the principal focus. This has the double benefit of restoring magnification and reducing the accommodative effort required to focus the divergent light from the image.

Self-evidently, aspheric and best form lenses will give better image quality than spherical lenses. Equally obviously, the power, diameter and field of view of a magnifier are related. The greater the power, the smaller the diameter and the more restricted the field of view. This gives rise to probably the most commonly heard complaint from patients using magnifiers – 'I can see really well with it, the letters are very clear, but I can only see a couple of words at a time. I want one just like this – only bigger!'

It should be obvious by now that the way in which a hand or stand lens is used has almost as much bearing on the final magnification and vision achieved as does the manufacturer's rating stamped on the unit.

The practitioner should always take the trouble to examine and look through the various magnifiers available and endeavour to arrive at a comparatively impartial assessment of their relative performance. Only the inexperienced accept the manufacturer's descriptions uncritically!

5.2   Survey of currently available hand and stand magnifiers

5.2.1   Hand magnifiers (loupes).

Units may be conveniently subdivided into:

(1)   Low-medium magnification, non-illuminated units.
(2)   Illuminated hand lenses.
(3)   High powered loupes and folding pocket units.

Some general observations apply to all hand lenses. In all except equiconvex forms the magnifier should be held so that the more curved surface is towards the eye. This has the effect of slightly reducing the distortional aberration.

All manufacturers have adopted the maximum magnification formula for rating their lenses.

$$\text{Magnification} = \frac{F}{4} + 1$$

Thus lens power F = +3.00, f = 33⅓ cm magnification 1.75×
                    F = +10.00, f = 10 cm magnification 3.5×
                    F = +20.00, f = 5 cm magnification 6×

(1)   Low-medium power, non-illuminated lenses

Small pocket folding or slide-out magnifiers (Fig. 5.7)

Specification range:

Magnification: 3× to 6×

Lens diameter: (Ø) 25–60 mm.

Lens form: generally biconvex plastics. Eschenbach double lens slide-out unit is in plano-convex form which makes an aplanatic system when both lenses are in use.

Comments: The integral cover helps to protect the lens surface from scratching and the compact size and inexpensive nature of the majority of the units renders them useful for issuing to patients in addition to their main near unit. It is impractical to carry large bulky magnifiers around, and impossible to wander round a large store wearing telescopic reading glasses for example. These little lenses, although generally too small for prolonged close work, can be easily slipped into a pocket and prove very useful for one-off, short duration tasks, such as checking prices, instruction labels, reading forms in the bank or post office, etc.

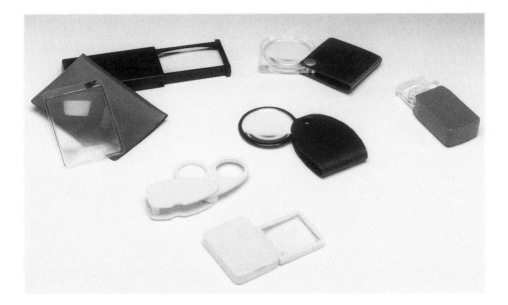

Fig. 5.7 Examples of small pocket-sized folding or slide-out magnifiers. Fresnel lenses, 3×, Ø 45 × 70 mm; Waltex sliding magnifier 2×, Ø 30 × 60 mm; folding magnifiers, 3.5×, Ø 45 and 50 mm; Beck double slide-out loupe, 3×/3× Ø 25 × 25 mm; COIL Duplex lens, 3.5×/5×, Ø 25 mm: COIL 5100 folding lens, 3.2×, Ø 33 × 29 mm. Available from most magnifier suppliers.

Larger aperture, non-aspheric lenses (Fig. 5.8)

Specification range:

Magnification: 2× to 4.4×

Lens diameter: Ø 40−120 mm round, 80 × 40 mm to 120 × 55 mm rectangular.

Lens form: biconvex lenses in clear or coloured plastics, chrome or gold metal mountings.

Comments: Standard lenses are inexpensive and reasonably lightweight although the larger ones are obviously on the bulky side. It is also possible to purchase more expensive 'decorative, fashion magnifiers'. Eschenbach also do a very neat, chrome or gold plated 3.5× Ø 45 mm glass biconvex lens on a chain which although not really appropriate for supply on a free-loan NHS basis is an attractive way of providing a modest amount of magnification for use in more formal social surroundings.

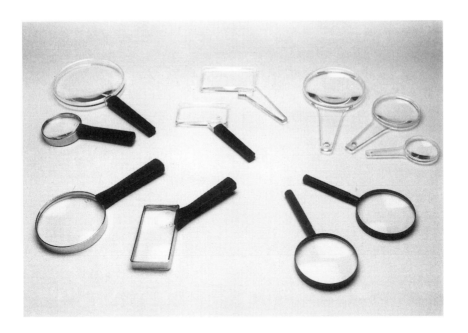

Fig. 5.8 Examples of large aperture, non-aspheric, low power hand lenses. Eschenbach 2641, 2×, Ø 120 mm, 2.5× Ø 80 × 40 mm, 2610 2×, Ø 90 × 50 mm, COIL Windsor range: 2.3× Ø 98 mm, 2.6× Ø 70 mm, 4.4× Ø 48 mm; COIL Victoria lenses 2.25× Ø 82 mm; Eschenbach 2320 lenses, 2× with 5× bifocal insert Ø 100 × 50 mm, 2× Ø 100 mm, 3× Ø 65 mm. Available from COIL, Associated Optical and most magnifier suppliers.

Aspheric and aplanatic lens forms (Fig. 5.9)

Specification range:
Magnification: 3× to 6×
Lens: Ø 50−80 mm round; 70 × 50 mm to 100 × 75 mm rectangular.
Lens form: aspheric or aplanatic lenses in plastics or metal mounts.
Comments: much improved image quality. More expensive. Included in this category are the so-called hand/stand magnifiers with a hinged handle and metal legs which can be folded away inside the lens mounting if not required, or swung down to form a slightly wobbly support and distance guide for the lens. The 'front' legs are adjustable to enable the lens to be tilted relative to the plane of the paper, if desired. Adjustable stands are available (Fig. 5.9.) which enable a hand lens to be positioned over or in front of an object, leaving both hands free.

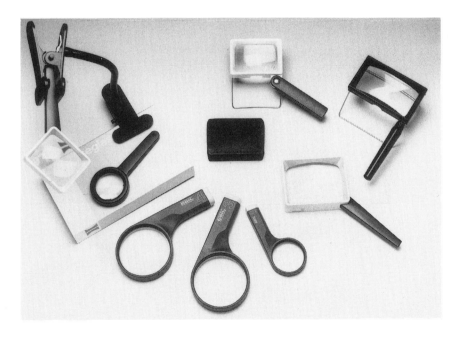

Fig. 5.9 Examples of aspheric and aplanatic hand and hand/stand lenses. Eschenbach units: table clamp (ref. 1600) with 2660, 4× Ø 70 × 55 mm lens, 2650 6× Ø 50 mm, hand/stand units with case, 2030 3× Ø 78 × 55 mm, 2036 2.75× Ø 100 × 50 mm, 2665 hand lens 3× Ø 100 × 75 mm; COIL aspheric hand magnifiers: 5206 6× Ø 50 mm, 5203 3× Ø 81 mm, 5204 4× Ø 80 mm.

5.2.2   **Illuminated hand lenses** (Fig. 5.10)

Specification range:

Magnification: 2.5× to 6×

Lens diameter: Ø 30−80 mm

Comments: the range of internally illuminated hand lenses is small and the light output limited by the need to keep the bulk and weight of the unit as low as possible. Batteries need replacing frequently since their life is limited, but the magnifier can be used quite satisfactorily in its non-illuminated form if necessary.

An interesting development from Eschenbach is their 'Super-Lite'; a 5 W fluorescent tube in a white plastics tubular mounting which clips onto some of their standard magnifier range. The unit with its 2 m of cable and transformer, gives a very high light output, is shadow free and has a life of approximately 5000 hours. The brightness can be adjusted.

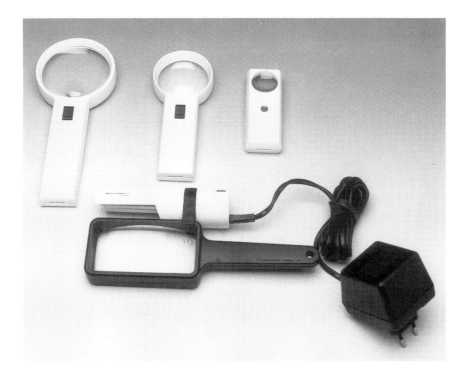

Fig. 5.10 Illuminated hand lenses. Eschenbach units: 2.5× with 5× bifocal insert, Ø 80 mm, 4× Ø 60 mm, 6× Ø 30 mm, all powered by two 1.5 V batteries. 'Super-Lite' mains powered 5 W fluorescent light attached to 2650 3× aspheric lens.

5.2.3   High powered loupes and pocket magnifiers (Fig. 5.11)

Specification range:
Magnification: 7× to 20×
Lens diameter: Ø 14−20 mm
Lens form: aplanatic glass or plastics lenses.
Comments: extremely limited field owing to the very small diameter, high powered lenses involved. Used as an 'occasional' aid when very high magnification is required for specific tasks. For example, a child studying geography might need a very powerful lens for the precise detail on Ordnance Survey maps, although other more general near vision requirements were satisfied with far less magnification.

5.3   Stand magnifiers

The extensive range of lenses available can be conveniently grouped into:

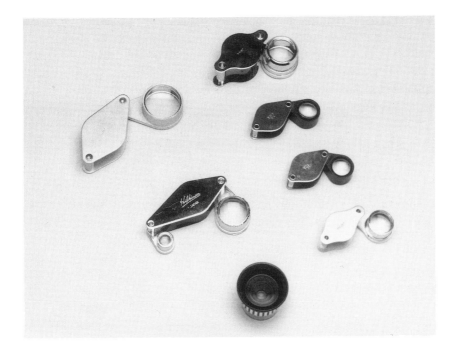

Fig. 5.11 Examples of high powered loupes and pocket magnifiers. Ruper 10× Ø 20 mm, Ruper 6× Ø 25 mm, 20× Ø 15 mm, 15× Ø 15 mm, Ruper double unit 10×/20×, 12× Ø 16 mm, Peak 30× Ø 7 mm. Available from all major magnifier suppliers.

(1) Non-illuminated low powered units, up to approximately 4× magnification:
     fixed stand units,
     variable, flexible stand and suspended magnifiers,
     bar magnifiers,
     flat-field magnifiers.

(2) Non-illuminated medium-high power magnifiers and loupes.

(3) Illuminated units

     fixed stand units,
     variable flexible stand units.

The overwhelming majority of stand units are rated on the maximum magnification system. However, as previously indicated, manufacturers use different stand heights for lenses with the same maximum magnification rating. Units with identical magnification stamped on the mounting may in reality give rise to significantly different magnification and aberration effects. Fig. 5.12 illustrates this for two identical diameter (50 mm), identically rated 6× units: the COIL 4206 and Eschenbach 2626 magnifiers. It can be seen that the magnification, field and aberration effects differ considerably for the two lenses.

All stand lenses require the use of accommodation and/or reading spectacles. The fact that individual variation in accommodation and preferred object/lens/eye positioning markedly affect the magnification produced, necessitates the assumption of a standard method of use. For comparative purposes it will be assumed that the magnified virtual image is formed in the focal plane of the user's spectacles. For convenience this distance is assumed to be 25 cm to eliminate the need to recalculate the manufacturer's lens ratings.

5.3.1   Non-illuminated low powered units

Most lenses in this category are large enough to permit binocular viewing with the possibility of writing under the lens.

Fixed stand lenses (Fig. 5.13)
Specification range:
Magnification: 1.7× to 4×
Lens: Ø 40−100 mm round; 50 × 30 to 140 × 100 mm rectangular.
Lens form: low magnification, large lenses are usually biconvex plastics, 3× to 4× range usually aspheric design.
Comments: the large stand lenses are appropriate when the degree of impairment is not too severe, but the person would have difficulty in maintaining a hand lens at the correct working distance, either because of hand tremor or possibly from a lack of understanding, in the case of a younger child. Also, as it is possible to

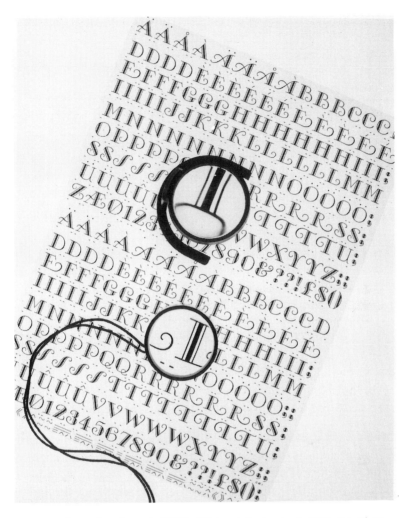

Fig. 5.12 Image formation through COIL 4206 and Eschenbach 2626 6×, Ø 50 mm stand lenses, illustrating the effect of varying lens form and stand height.

get a pen or finger under the lens to draw attention to a specific letter or object, they are also particularly useful for teachers of visually handicapped pupils.

A stand lens might well be the unit of choice for someone engaged in manual activity e.g. assembly work, knitting, model-making, etc. who can manage to see the task itself but needs periodically to read instructions or the pattern and so on. The lens sits on the instruction sheet which is constantly in focus, and is 'nudged' along as required without the person having to disengage one hand from the task.

The major difficulties with stand lenses are a tendency for the mounting to

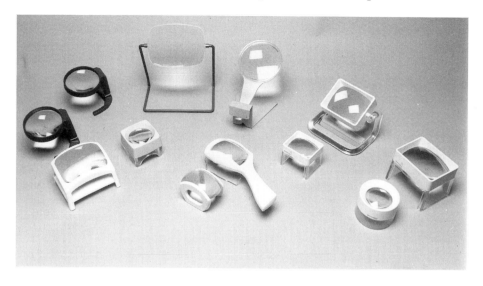

Fig. 5.13   Lower power fixed stand magnifiers, 1.7× to 4× magnification. Selection of stand magnifiers: *back row, from left*: COIL 5213 3× Ø 81 mm, 5214 4× Ø 80 mm, Clear view (5855) 1.7× Ø 140 × 100 mm, Handstand (5291) 2.3× Ø 98 mm; Eschenbach 2622 3× Ø 100 × 75 mm variable angle lens with optional 2602 bar mag, 2623 3 × Ø 100 × 75 mm. *Front row*: Schweizer 'Twin' 911 lens, 3× Ø 100 × 75 mm with removable lower lens 2.5×; total unit 4.5× Ø 70 × 40 mm, 321 4× Ø 60 mm; LHP 'The Style' hand/stand lens 3.7× Ø 85 × 45 mm, LHP Compacte 3.7× Ø 75 × 40 mm; Eschenbach 2625 4× Ø 79 × 55 mm, 2627 4× Ø 60 mm.

cast a shadow on the page and the need to look at right angles through the lens in order to minimise aberrations and utilise the full field of view. Light direction can sometimes be a problem and the user may have to pick up and angle the 'magnifier plus print' unit in order to obtain an adequate view through the lens. If the magnifier is flat on a desk one has to bend forward and peer over the top of the lens, finishing the task roundshouldered and with backache (Figs 5.14 and 5.20). A few lens designs feature a swivel attachment for the lens so that the plane of the lens can be altered although the stand itself is fixed. The LHP 26 lens is a double unit with the upper lens fixed in the mounting but inclined approximately 15° to the horizontal.

Variable flexible stand and suspended chest magnifiers (Fig. 5.15)

Specification range:
Magnification: 1.7× to 4×
Lens: Ø 60 mm round up to 140 × 100 mm rectangular. Arm length 320 mm (1.7× unit) to 150 mm (4× unit).
Comments: some units have the option of a table base or a clamp fitting. Low magnification, not really portable, but relatively inexpensive and ideal for

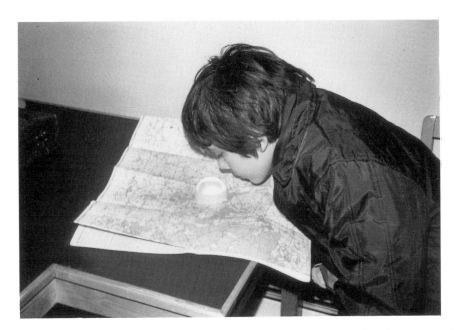

Fig. 5.14 Postural problems association with stand lenses. Map reading in a geography lesson with a flat field magnifier.

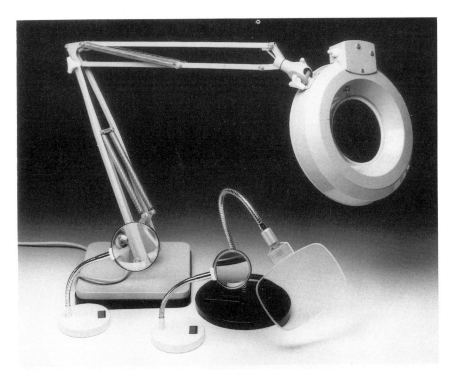

Fig. 5.15 Examples of flexible stand magnifiers. FEMO illuminated magnifier, basic unit 1.75 × Ø 108 mm, circular 22 W fluorescent tube, clamp or table base. (Available from Viking Optical Ltd, Newbold & Bulford Ltd.) Non-illuminated Eschenbach 2.5× Ø 80 mm and 4× Ø 60 mm units and COIL FlexiMag 1.7× Ø 140 × 100 mm.

writing and manual tasks. It is easy to get supplementary lighting onto the task if required.

Suspended chest magnifiers are again low powered, inexpensive units which leave both hands free for sewing, knitting, etc. Useful for those who only require minimal magnification. They do have the irritating, though obviously unavoidable, tendency to bounce around somewhat as their users breathe.

Bar magnifiers (Fig. 5.16)

Specification range:
Magnification: 1.5× in one direction
Lens: Ø 120 × 25 mm to 350 × 35 mm
Lens form: plano-cylindrical lenses. Used flat on the page parallel to the print lines, they will magnify the height of the letters. Made of plastics or Plexiglas, the underside being either slightly concave or having a narrow flange along the edge to minimise scratching.
Comments: despite their low magnification, bar magnifiers have a greater appli-

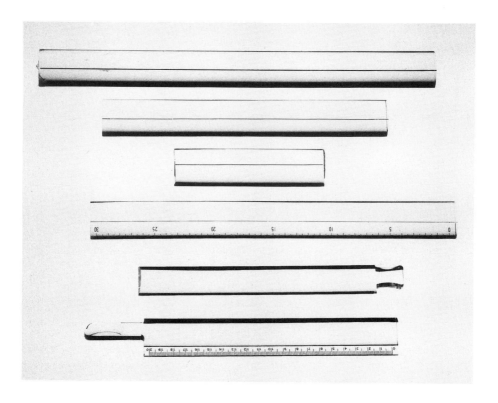

Fig. 5.16 Bar magnifiers. Eschenbach 2609 Ø 350 × 35 mm, 2608 Ø 250 × 35 mm, 2602 Ø 128 × 35 mm all with red guide line; Newbold & Bulford 491 200 Ø 310 × 25 mm, with guide line and scale; LHP LR200 Ø 200 × 30 mm with scale (Specialist Optical Source).

cation than might at first appear to be the case. They have excellent light-gathering properties and produce completely distortion-free magnification. The size can be selected for the particular paper size in use. The longest bar magnifier which is 35 cm long will cover the full width of computer paper. Some have a measuring scale at the side, others a red line engraved along the centre of the underside of the lens. This guide line is a particularly useful tracking device to help correlate entries in columns of figures spread across a page such as would be encountered in account books, bank statements, VDU and computer printout sheets.

The large size and normal working distance again enable comfortable binocular viewing to be maintained.

Flat-field magnifiers (Fig. 5.17)

Specification range:
Magnification approximately 1.8× at 30–40 cm viewing distance.
Lens: Ø 40–90 mm diameter
Lens form: solid hemispherical planoconvex glass or plastics lenses. Used flat on the page, they have either a plastics mounting or a slightly concave base to

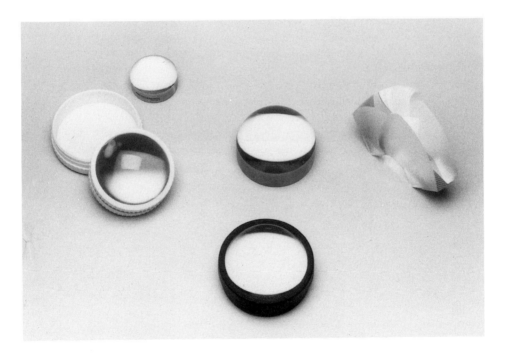

Fig. 5.17 Flat field magnifiers. Hemispherical lenses Ø 40 to 90 mm available from Schweizer and Eschenbach. LHP T4 'Hedgehog' magnifier (Specialist Optical Source) is a clever modification of the flat field/bar magnifier principle in which the base is shaped to enable it to fit into the curved spine of a book.

reduce scratching. Lenses without the plastics mounting have a dull, frosted rim for ease of handling and to limit distracting internal reflections.

Comments: optically similar to bar magnifiers, they have unrivalled light-gathering properties. The hemispherical surface collects all the light incident upon it and concentrates it onto the working plane. They are best used in good, general diffuse room illumination. Strong directional light sources can cause annoying surface reflections. It has a distortion-free field of view. Manufacturers claim it is possible to achieve up to 6× magnification with flat-field lenses by utilising a short eye-magnifier distance and exerting a significant amount of accommodation. Feasible for children, but not for elderly patients.

5.3.2   Non-illuminated medium to high power magnifiers and loupes (Fig. 5.18)

Specification range:
Magnification: 6× to 20× in 'conventional' stand lenses, 8× to 22× in small loupes.

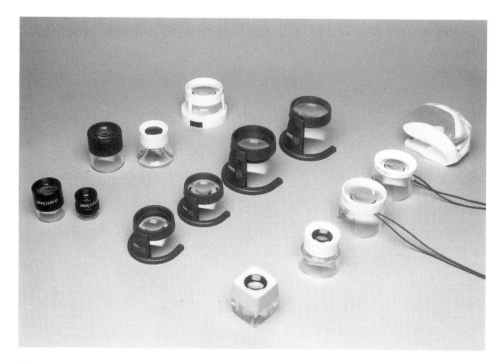

Fig. 5.18 Non-illuminated, medium to high power stand magnifiers. *Left row*: Block magnifier 10× Ø 50 mm; Wahl 10× Ø 26 mm, Wahl 8× Ø 24 m; Peak loupes 10× Ø 25 mm, 22× Ø 15 mm; *Middle row*: COIL 4206 6× Ø 50 mm, 4208 8× Ø 44 mm, 4210 10× Ø 36 mm, 4212 12× Ø 34 mm; *Right row*: LHP26 Sphero-Cyl, double lens, ≏ 4×, Ø 70 × 20 mm Eschenbach 2624 8× Ø 35 mm, 2626 6× Ø 50 mm, 1153 8× Ø 25 mm; Beck 8× Ø 23 mm.

Lens: Ø 50 mm to 20 mm

Comments: the range of units is comparatively restricted since the small lens diameters and short focal lengths start to introduce illumination problems. For this reason, many higher powered units are produced in illuminated form. The block magnifier is an interesting attempt to utilise the flat-field magnifiers hemispherical light-gathering properties within a two lens system to produce a high powered unit (10×) with a larger aperture and thus potentially greater visual field. COIL have recently extended their range of non-illuminated stand magnifiers to include adjustable focus units, of 15× and 20× magnification. High powered units are effectively monocular in use.

5.3.3 Illuminated units (Fig. 5.19)

Fixed stand units

Specification range:

Magnification: 3× to 15× round; 2.75× to 3× rectangular

Lens: Ø 80−20 mm round, 104 × 75 to 100 × 50 mm rectangular.

Mountings of Schweizer and Eschenbach units are white/cream, COIL units are steel blue and Peak lenses have black surrounds.

Comments: Peak units and one or two cheaper torch magnifiers are only available with standard battery operation. The majority of the better quality units have mains or rechargeable battery transformer options. In addition an increasing number of units may be obtained with halogen bulbs.

Standard tungsten bulbs are 2.5 V/250 mA in comparison to the 5.2 V/500 mA rating of halogen bulbs. It is important to be clear which type of bulb is in a given unit. Halogen bulbs produce a much brighter, whiter (i.e. less yellow) light and have a much longer life than tungsten bulbs but they are mains only, require a specialised transformer and cannot usually be battery operated. The magnifier, bulb and power unit should all be obtained from the same source to ensure safety and compatibility of the complete unit.

Schweizer lenses and some of the Eschenbach units have mountings shaped to hold the lens at an angle to provide a slightly easier, more natural viewing position. The COIL lenses can be tilted as desired by the patient.

The COIL illuminated range does allow examination of solid objects since the lens extends beyond the end of the light housing. It is of restricted value, however, because of the small diameter and short focal length of the lenses involved. The Eschenbach clip-on fluorescent light (See section [5.2.2] can be attached to the large 3× swivel stand lens (reference 2622). Since the lens can be rotated through 360° it gives the option of an illuminated, magnified view of rather larger 3D objects which can be inserted and manipulated under the lens. Limited writing is also possible. All other units are designed to be positioned flat on the page.

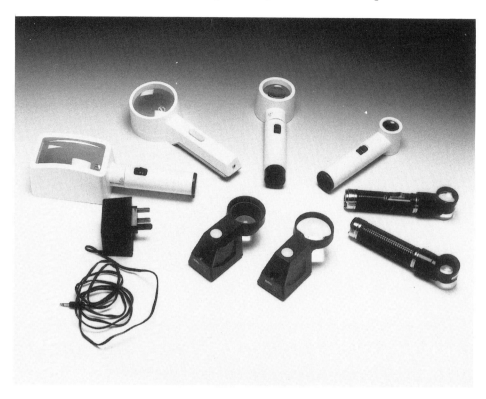

Fig. 5.19 Fixed stand illuminated units. Selected samples from Eschenbach, Schweizer, Peak and COIL ranges. Peak units are only available with standard battery handles. Most others have battery or mains options and many are available with halogen bulbs. Shown in the illustration: Eschenbach 3× Ø 100 × 50 mm, 4× Ø 60 mm, 7× Ø 30 mm; Schweizer 3.5× Ø 75 mm; Peak 10× and 15× units; COIL 6× Ø 50 mm and 12× Ø 34 mm units.

Illuminated units are particularly useful for elderly people where media changes are a significant part of their visual problem. The internal illumination frequently enables the magnification level to be reduced, with consequent improvement in field.

The limited field of view is still a problem, but since there is no longer any need to worry about shadowing, or the necessity of getting adequate external illumination onto the print, patients often seem more prepared to bring the lens closer to their eyes, almost into the spectacle plane at times, thus benefiting from the resultant field improvement induced.

The major drawbacks of such magnifiers generally relate to their bulk and the need to keep replacing batteries or restrict use to the vicinity of a power point. Sometimes design weaknesses such as fragility of switches, or the difficulty of opening the housing to change batteries are a cause of major dissatisfaction. It can be quite difficult for a normally sighted, dextrous person to 'get at' the batteries in some units. For an arthritic, partially sighted individual it can be impossible.

Variable flexible stand units (Fig. 5.15)

Specification range:
Magnification: 1.75× to 2× basic units, auxiliary lenses to 2.75×, 3.5× and 3.75×,
Lens: Ø 100−128 mm diameter.
Lens form and illumination: glass lenses. Illumination currently from 60 W tungsten bulbs, 7 W or 11 W straight, or 22 W circular fluorescent tubes. All mains-operated with transformer.
Comments: available with clamp or table bases and flexible or spring-tension jointed arms. They are heavy, non-portable and expensive but can solve specific problems when nothing else is appropriate − for example, something requiring extensive manipulative room plus a good light such as industrial inspection procedures, crafts, and some school subjects such as biology.

5.4   Summary

Hand and stand magnifiers are a quick, relatively inexpensive way of providing 'instant' magnification and are the unit of choice for very many people. Those who require magnification for comparatively short periods of time, for an assortment of activities through the day, or those who reject the short working distance of head-borne units may use a hand or stand lens very happily.

Hand tremor predisposes towards stand lenses, and media and lighting problems towards internally illuminated units. The fact that a magnifier can be supplied and exchanged from stock renders it useful for patients with rapidly varying visual problems.

Some diabetic patients, patients with active inflammatory conditions, short-term problems while awaiting or immediately after surgery are all particularly suited to the rapid availability and interchangeability of hand or stand magnifiers.

It is very much an area in which the practitioner must offer guidance, then be prepared to stand back and let the patients experiment and 'do their own thing' with the various lenses!

Accommodation permitting, moving the lens-object unit closer to the eyes increases the field of view and magnification by superimposing relative distance magnification effects onto the angular magnification effects of the lens. Those with active accommodation have more options, but even very elderly people have considerable flexibility in the choice of object to lens, and lens to eye positioning to give optimum vision.

Higher powered lenses are invariably circular, but at lower powers there is often a choice between aspheric and non-aspheric, circular or rectangular designs.

Added to this is the 'with or without spectacles' dimension. Hyperopes may prefer to use a higher powered unit without glasses, rather than a lower powered option which necessitates juggling with distance and reading glasses plus magnifier all the time. Myopes also may well find that some magnifiers give a more satisfactory level of performance if used without spectacles. For other lenses, removing glasses makes things worse.

The permutations are so many and varied that only an inexperienced (or very foolhardy) practitioner would give a patient categorical instructions on 'How to use this magnifier'. Almost invariably the patient will get better results by doing something quite different. No two patients are quite the same in the way they respond to these or any other types of optical aid. They have to have advice, but the range and variety of solutions that evolve is an aspect that adds considerable interest to work with visually impaired people (Fig. 5.20).

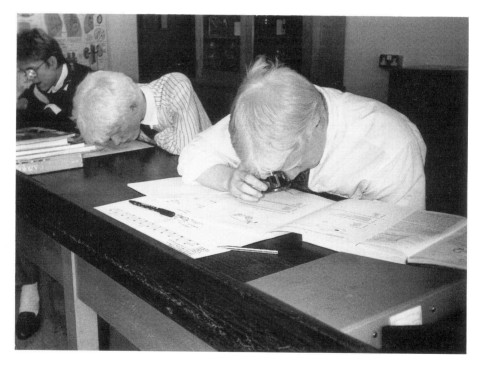

Fig. 5.20 Albino pupil using COIL 6× stand lens in the spectacle plane, like a microscopic spectacle lens without the frame.

Questions

1 What do you understand by the term nominal magnification?
   (See section [5.1.2].)

2 Explain the concept of the 'least distance of distinct vision'.
   (See section [5.1.2].)

3 What is maximum magnification?
   (See section [5.1.3].)

4 What problems arise at present as a result of the absence of standard policy
   concerning magnifier magnification and power specification?
   (See section [5.1.4].)

5 How does the object−lens separation affect:

   (a) The magnification produced

   (b) The need for distance or near spectacles on the part of the user?
   (See section [5.1.5].)

6 What factors influence the field of view obtained with a hand or stand lens?
   (See section [5.1.6].)

7 In general terms, how much magnification is available in conventional hand
   magnifiers?
   Can one obtain illuminated hand magnifiers?
   (See section [5.2.1].)

8 Similarly to question 7, for stand magnifiers, how much magnification is
   available? (See section [5.3].)
   Many stand magnifiers are internally illuminated. What are the advantages
   and pitfalls of halogen bulbs compared to the more familiar tungsten bulbs?
   (See section [5.3.3].)

9 What are bar magnifiers and flat-field magnifiers?
   (See section [5.3.1(3)].)

10 What type of unit might you consider for examination of three dimensional
    objects?
    (See section [5.3.1] and [5.3.3(2)].)

CHAPTER 6

Near Vision: Head-borne and Spectacle Mounted Units

Many near vision tasks require the use of both hands and necessitate the provision of some form of head-borne or spectacle mounted unit.

6.1   Non-telescopic units

The terminology is confusing. 'Microscopic spectacles', 'near vision microscope', 'high add', 'magnifying spectacles', are all terms found in the literature to describe what are basically high plus lenses, worn in the spectacle plane.

6.1.1   Optical principles

The description of high plus lenses worn in the spectacle plane as 'magnifying' or 'microscopic' spectacles is misleading. It implies that magnification is achieved by optical means, angular magnification, whereas in reality magnification is the result of employing relative distance magnification principles.

Moving an object closer and closer to the eye creates a progressively larger retinal image. If the person has sufficient accommodation available, the enlarged retinal image will be focussed clearly. This is the 'built-in magnifier' situation which prevails with many visually impaired children. In the absence of adequate accommodation, a supplementary plus lens will be required to maintain an in-focus retinal image.

The closer the object is positioned relative to the eyes, the larger will be the retinal image (i.e. the greater the magnification) but the greater will be the accommodation and/or supplementary lens power to focus the resultant retinal image. Technically, the high plus lens is acting, not as an optical magnifier, but as 'artificial' accommodation!

Certain assumptions are necessary if we are to compare and contrast the various available units. It is assumed that the lens-power/object distance relationship is such that the object is positioned at the first principal focus (thin lens theory), or more correctly, in the front vertex focal plane of the lens. This produces parallel incident light at the eye, with theoretically zero accommodative demand.

In practice however, the amount of available accommodation does influence the magnification effects of all the various head-borne and spectacle mounted units. As with hand and stand magnifiers there is considerable variation in the object position selected, with resultant variation in magnification, field of view and depth of field, for any given unit.

The baseline magnification is however established by comparing the actual angular subtense of an object, with the angular subtense of the same object positioned at the 'least distance of distinct vision' reference distance. Manufacturers adopt the 25 cm reference distance. For example, an object at 10 cm distance subtends 2.5× the angle subtended by the same object at 25 cm distance. Since 10D accommodation or a +10D FVP supplementary lens would be needed to focus the object at 10 cm range, the lens in the spectacle plane is said to have a 2.5× magnification effect. This is equal to the nominal magnification of the lens.

Thus, assuming the object is positioned in the front vertex focal plane of the lens, the nominal magnification equates exactly with the relative distance magnification effects. Hence it is much more convenient, although technically incorrect, to talk of the 'magnification' of a high plus lens in the spectacle plane in terms of its power and nominal magnification.

Manufacturers invariably adopt the $\dfrac{F}{4}$ nominal magnification basis to specify the magnification of integral spectacle mounted units. However, the uncertainty regarding the precise nature of F applies with equal force to spectacle mounted units as it does to hand and stand lenses. Such units comprise thick lenses and accurate comparison is only possible if the equivalent powers are known and nominal magnification correctly designated in terms of $\dfrac{F_e}{4}$

6.1.2 Comparison of non-telescopic with telescopic spectacle mounted units

Advantages of non-telescopic units

(1) Relatively large field of view.
    Field of view and working distance are inversely related. A single lens in the spectacle plane will always have the optimum field of view for any given magnification compared with the equivalent near telescopic unit.
(2) Lightweight and relatively inconspicuous.
    Headband units are naturally more bulky, but high plus plastics lenses in a conventional spectacle frame are neat, light and inconspicuous. They may be dispensed in full-aperture, half-eye or bifocal form.

Disadvantages of non-telescopic units

(1)   Short working distance.
(2)   Difficulties associated with illumination.
(3)   Aberrations.
(4)   Binocularity/convergence considerations.

(1)   Short working distance

As we have seen, the working distance is directly related to the magnification and to the power of the spectacle lens.

i.e.:

> +10.00DS, WD 10 cm, nominal magnification 2.5×.
> +20.00DS, WD 5 cm, nominal magnification 5×.

Quite small movements of the object either side of the principal focus will give rise to substantial convergence or divergence of the light reaching the eye. The greater the available accommodation the more the eye is able to compensate for object movement, and the greater will be the effective depth of field. An elderly patient with limited accommodation has a correspondingly limited depth of field and object positioning becomes very critical.

Although the hands are free the short working distance limits the range of tasks that can be performed with this type of unit.

(2)   Difficulties associated with illumination

The need to hold objects close to the eyes frequently produces illumination problems. Young eyes with clear media generally cope reasonably well. Those with central congenital cataracts may ironically find the lower light levels and consequent pupil dilation beneficial.

Weale (1963) considers that as a normal consequence of ageing, in the absence of any additional ocular pathology, a 60 year old retina receives only one third of the light incident on a 20 year old retina. Many elderly patients have significant media opacities superimposed on the normal age-related effects. Obtaining sufficient object illumination for such patients using high plus lenses can be a considerable problem.

(3)   Aberrations

Bennett (1975) considers oblique astigmatism and distortion to be the major optical aberrations limiting performance of high powered spherical surfaces. Aspheric plastics lenses should be used whenever possible. Up to +20.00D the aspheric lens ranges primarily intended for aphakic correction should be used, e.g. Omega and Rodenstock Perfastar lenses.

Above that power the Igard Hyperocular range (4× to 12×) of biconvex aspheric lenticular lenses is likely to give the best optical performance in single vision lens form. From approximately 10× magnification there are some optical advantages in having a doublet or triplet compound lens unit, e.g. Keeler LVA 9. The additional bulk, however, resembles a telescopic unit, so eliminating one of the normal advantages of this category of unit.

(4) Binocularity/convergence considerations

Many visually impaired people have a large difference between the acuities of their two eyes. Prescribed aids are likely to be for monocular use. If, however, an attempt is to be made to keep the person binocular, the short working distances of these high add, microscopic, systems will impose severe convergence demands on the oculo-motor system. It will be necessary to relieve this convergence demand with base − in prism.

6.1.3   Estimation of base-in prism requirement

There are a number of differing calculations and 'rules-of-thumb' that have been advocated to determine the amount of prism required.

(1)   Lebensohn's rule (Lebensohn, 1949)

The difference between the distance and near interpupillary distances (PD) is determined by dividing the distance interpupillary distance in millimetres by the reading distance, in inches, plus one.

Example
Emmetropic patient. Distance PD 66 mm, using +8.00D add.
At working distance 12.5 cm = 5 inches.
Thus $66 \div (5 + 1) = 11$.
If the near optical centre (OC) were set at $66 - 11 = 55$ mm the visual axes would be coincident with the near OC when the spectacles were in use, i.e. the patient must converge by 5½ mm in each eye to achieve binocular single vision through the glasses in the absence of relieving prism. This convergence, 5½ mm on a +8.00D lens $\equiv 4.4^{\Delta}$ each eye. It would necessary to work 4.4^{Δ}B. in each eye, effective at the distance PD 66, to enable the eyes to view the near object without the need to converge.

(2)   Fonda's 'rule-of-thumb' (Fonda, 1978)

This suggests that lenses should be decentred in by 1 mm per dioptre add each eye.

Example

The same emmetropic patient, distance PD 66, +8.00D add

Gives: 8 mm decentration EE on +8.00D lens = 6.4^{\triangle} each eye.

Total 12.8^{\Delta} for spectacles as a whole, effective at 66 mm

(3) Jackson & Silver (Visual Disability Part 4, 1983)

Jackson & Silver point out that every dioptre of focussing for near vision, whether by accommodation or lens addition, is associated with a 1 metre angle (MA) convergence movement by each eye (Fig. 6.1). In order to maintain binocular single vision, a person viewing an object 25 cm away must exert 4 MA convergence with each eye. An object at 12.5 cm range requires 8 MA convergence each eye, etc. The size of the MA depends not only on the viewing distance, but also on the subject's PD and so is a variable quantity.

MA measurements can be easily translated into more familiar prism dioptre units:

Convergence of each eye (in prism dioptres) = (Number of MA) \times (½ PD in cm)

Example 1: Normal person, PD 66 mm, reading at 25 cm range. Convergence each eye = 4 \text{ MA} \times 3.3 = 13.2^{\Delta}; binocular = 26.4^{\Delta}.

Example 2: Same person, PD 66 mm, now reading with +8.00D add at 12.5 cm range.
Monocular convergence = 8 \text{ MA} \times 3.3 = 26.4^{\triangle}; binocular =

52.8^{\Delta}.

Thus these different viewpoints on the same problem produce widely differing recommendations regarding the amount of prism required. For the example patient, all recommendations are well below the actual 26.4^{\Delta} additional convergence required to retain binocular single vision when changing from 25 cm to 12.5 cm viewing distance.

In theory, it is impossible to overdo the base-in prism. The more the better. In reality, the ocular system copes remarkably well without large amounts of prism. Furthermore, incorporating large amounts of prism increases the weight, thickness and chromatic aberration of the lens and may generate considerable manufacturing problems. The nasal edge lens thickness resulting from the base-in prism may also produce frame fitting or cosmetic appearance complications. If the material thickness has been glazed predominantly behind the rim to enhance the cosmetic appearance it is inclined to dig into the nose or inner canthus. If it is glazed to the front of the rim, the frame can be fitted nice and close to the eyes, but the patient is inclined to object to the 'ugly thick glasses'.

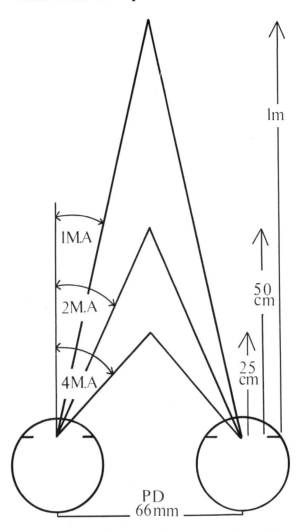

Fig. 6.1 Convergence considerations in terms of metre angles. Every dioptre of focussing for near vision, by accommodation or supplementary lens, is associated with one metre angle of convergence movement by each eye.

The uncertainty over what is really required seems to render complicted calculations rather pointless. A lot of practitioners, myself included, tend to use the easier 'guestimate' of $1^\Delta B$ in each eye for every dioptre add, effective at the distance PD; or $1^\Delta B$ in each eye for every dioptre add over +3.00D, effective at the near PD. (Both 'guestimates' amount to roughly the same thing.) This seems to work quite acceptably from a clinical standpoint.

6.1.4   Dispensing considerations

(1)   Back vertex distance

All spectacle-mounted units should be fitted as close to the eyes as possible:

- To maximise the field of view.
- To gain maximum benefit from base-in prism.

  Assuming the eye has some accommodation available, the patient is likely to use it to improve the depth of field of the object and to increase magnification.

$$F_{eq} = F_1 + F_2 - dF_1F_2$$

where
  F_{eq} = equivalent power 2 lens system in air.
  F_1 = power spectacle lens
  F_2 = accommodation used
   d = separation (mm) between lenses (effectively the BVD).

Bailey (1980) has shown that when d is small, the term dF_1F_2 can be ignored, and F_{eq} of the spectacle/accommodation system can be considered to be the sum of the two component parts.

   The closer the magnifying spectacle lens is placed to the eye, the truer this approximation becomes.

(2)   Centration

Centration considerations for binocular units and supplementary prism have already been discussed. Monocular unit orders should indicate ½PD measurements based on the patient's near PD for an orthodox 30 cm-ish reading position.

   I find that a lifetime's habit of holding print approximately symmetrically in front of their face stays with people even when reading monocularly. Those who have had normal vision almost invariably cope more comfortably with short working distance monocular vision if the basic eye position is slightly convergent. The position of the near vision point of the lens in the frame should therefore correspond with the visual axis in this comfortable 'normal' starting position. The oculo-motor scanning movements are then more natural.

   The lazy habit of getting the lens glazed to the geometrical centre of the rim usually results in the lens being decentred out, relative to the visual axis, introducing a sort of 'abnormal head posture' effect as the person attempts to line up the book, the lens and their eye.

6.1.5   Magnification rating

As we have seen, non-telescopic integral spectacle mounted units are rated in terms of the nominal magnification. However, clip-on and headband units tend to be rated in terms of the maximum magnification (F/4 + 1).

Presumably manufacturers assume such units will be attached to, or worn over, reading spectacles, or that alternatively the person will employ accommodation. The magnification effect, as far as the user was concerned, *would* then be F/4 + 1 − a little misleading, nonetheless.

Fortunately, these are generally low power units which may be treated as thin lenses. If in doubt, lens powers may be measured on a focimeter without incurring undue error.

Practitioners who prefer to use longer 'least distance of distinct vision' principles must recalculate the manufacturer's rating for all units.

6.1.6   Summary of units available

Units available may be conveniently subdivided as follows:

(1)   Single vision lenses.
(2)   Compound spectacle magnifiers.
(3)   Half-eye and bifocal units.
(4)   Clip-on spectacle magnifiers.
(5)   Headband magnifiers.
(6)   Watchmakers' eyeglass-type units.

(1)   Single vision lenses (Fig. 6.2)

Magnification range available 2× to 12×. This is the design of unit which has the potential for the greatest field of view of any spectacle mounted device. It is appropriate for exclusively close range, near vision activity with minimal or no distance vision requirement. Some binocularity is possible at low magnifications with base-in prism, otherwise monocular units would be supplied. The poorer eye should be occluded or glazed with the distance R_x or an afocal lens. After demonstrating the alternatives the choice should be left to the patient. Some find the blurred vision from the poorer eye interferes with and degrades the quality of the magnified image. They benefit from occlusion of that eye. Others seem able to ignore the unwanted image when reading and like to have a normal lens in front of the eye such that they have a sense of the room around them when glancing up from the near vision task.

The occluding lens may be totally opaque plastics or a frosted or chavasse-type lens which is cosmetically preferable. Elasoplast, micropore or translucent

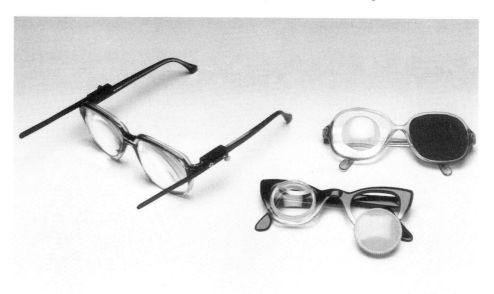

Fig. 6.2 High plus single vision spectacles. Rayner Raymag lenses with 'work posts' to stabilise object distance; COIL Hyperocular with occluder; Keeler LVA 10 lens with optional occluder, standard assembly.

stick-on Fablon are invaluable for a trial-run with patients who cannot make up their minds.

Low magnification requirements (up to approximately 4×, i.e. +16.00D) are most easily satisfied from standard aspheric aphakic lens ranges. Cyls up to 4.00D can then also be incorporated.

In the absence of a significant cylindrical element COIL Igard Hyperoculars are the best option for a single vision lens in the medium to high power range. These biconvex, aspheric lenticular lenses are available with quoted magnification 4×, 5×, 6×, 8×, 10×, 12×. Lens aperture and focal length (i.e. working distance) is related to the power ranging from 39 mm aperture, 57 mm focal length for the 4× unit to 29 mm aperture, 25 mm focal length for the 12× lens. These lenses may be dispensed into standard frames allowing for the normal constraints of blank size and centration.

The recently redesigned Rayner Raymag aspheric system provides a monocular 5×, 7×, or 9× lens fitted into either a Rayner standard frame or into a frame of the patient's choice. It is recommended that the frame has 'work support posts' fitted to minimise object movement.

Hyperocular and Raymag lenses, being preset fixed powers, cannot incorporate a cylindrical correction.

Keeler LVA 10 units (Fig. 6.2) on the other hand can be designed to incorporate the patient's refractive correction if required. The basic unit consists of a single aspheric lens, power 2× to 8× (excluding 7×). It may be fitted directly into the Keeler frame and secured with a metal locking ring, or it may be fitted into a flat glazed carrier lens with spacer, and then retained by a locking ring. This second system provides for a wide choice of frame with good control over the centration of the unit. Either assembly system allows powers to be freely interchanged as necessary. 6× and 8× units may be obtained with distance pieces attached. The spectacles are immediately more bulky but the greater object stability may be of benefit, especially to older patients with slight hand tremor.

A corrective lens in a cell can be fitted to the back of the unit. This adds to the size of the unit so if possible spherical ametropia should be incorporated into the basic magnification selected:

Thus:　Distance R_x +8.00D with 4× magnification = 6× magnification
　　　　Distance R_x −8.00D with 4× magnification = 2× magnification

(2)　　*Compound spectacle magnifiers* (Fig. 6.3)

Full lens units (i.e. purely near vision without any distance vision element) but made up of two or more lenses in a mounting to give the potential for greater magnification with better aberration control than would be possible with a single lens.

Bier-Hamblin compound reading units use a compound lens system over the whole of their magnification range from 2× to 12× and 15×. Cylindrical correction can be incorporated in all but the 15× unit. Magnification of 2× and 3× can be produced in binocular form with the manufacturer calculating the necessary prismatic adjustment relative to the patient's PD and the focal length of the unit. All other units should be used monocularly.

The high magnification compound spectacle magnifier units are at the top of the practical optical magnification range. Their very high powers result in focal lengths in the region of 2–3 cm from the end of the lens. Thus distance pieces are helpful and the great majority of the users also require in-built illumination. Occasionally young people with very clear media and/or media opacities or retinal lesions manage better without illumination.

Rayner's Raylight illuminated system is produced in a spectacle mounted design, 8×, 10×, 12×, 15×, with mains transformer or pocket battery power unit. Ametropia correction can easily be incorporated into the system.

The Keeler LVA9 series comprises five powers: 8×, 10×, 12×, 15× and 20×. It is available in spectacle mounted or hand-held, internally illuminated (via battery handle) or non-illuminated options. If non-illuminated, the opaque distance piece housing is replaced by a clear crystal housing. The position of the housing relative to the lens may be adjusted slightly to allow for small amounts of ametropia or

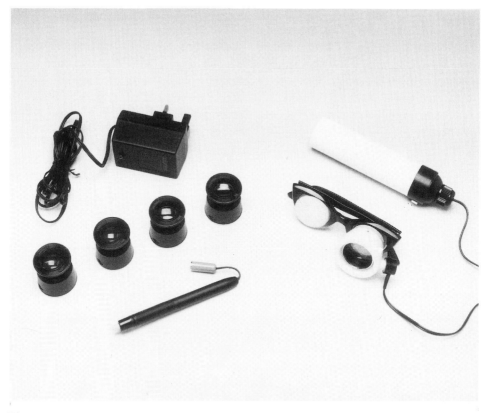

Fig. 6.3 Compound spectacle magnifiers. Rayner Raylight illuminated unit fitting set, Keeler LVA 9 series unit, spectacle mounted with battery handle.

accommodation but it is generally desirable to correct any underlying refractive error by means of a supplementary lens incorporated into the back of the unit.

Peak high magnification loupes can also be mounted in a spectacle frame to give a comparatively inexpensive non-illuminated unit.

Such high powered lenses inevitably severely restrict the field of view, to only three or four letters in some cases, so successful use requires a tremendous amount of motivation and a stubborn refusal to be beaten on the part of the patient. In addition the units are rather expensive. Realistically, therefore, their application will always be restricted. An LVA practitioner should nevertheless know about, and have access to such units, should the need arise (Fig. 6.4).

(3) Half-eye and bifocal units (Fig. 6.5)

This form of unit should be considered for people who require a rapid interchange of distance–near vision and to whom the short working distance is acceptable.

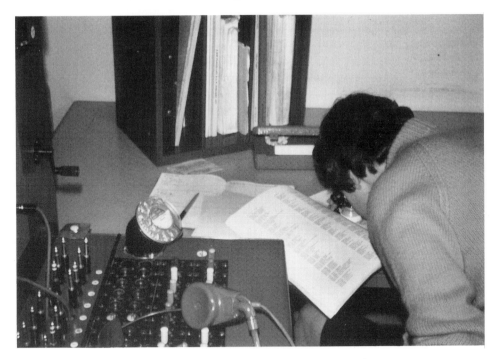

Fig. 6.4 Keeler LVA 9, 15× unit, in use to check telephone numbers.

Magnification available: 2× to 9×. Low to medium magnification: Standard prescription lenses with high add bifocal segments known as Sola LVA bifocals are CR39 moulded, front surface 25 mm round segment bifocals. Blank size 58 mm, Power −9.00 to +17.00D, cyls to −4DC, Add +4.00 to +16.00D. A smaller range of powers is available in a 38 mm segment lens.

This is a neat, inexpensive way of providing a modest amount of magnification for people with a significant amount of distance ametropia.

Emmetropic patients who only require this modest level of magnification (up to about +16.00D is practicable) may prefer prescription lenses fitted to any of the commercially available half-eye frames. Binocular vision with base-in prism or monocular viewing with an occluding or frosted lens again provides a neat, cosmetically acceptable, magnification device.

A small range of low powered, ready made half-eye units are available from the COIL, Eschenbach and Wahl product ranges.

Other options include the Bier-Hamblin compound reading unit which can be cut down and glazed into a purpose made half-eye with adjustable pads. This unit can also be ordered in Franklin split-bifocal form with a normal single vision distance portion and compound magnifying reading portion, fitted higher than a conventional bifocal.

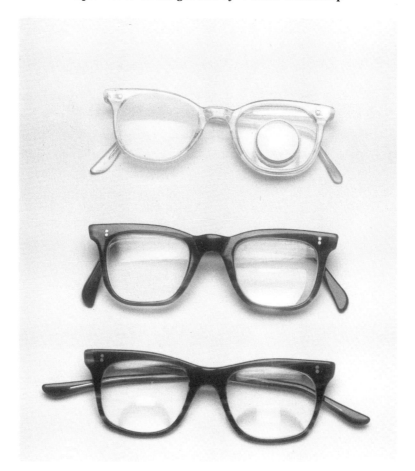

Fig. 6.5 Bifocal spectacles. Keeler LVA 12 (LE) with frosted RE; cemented high plus D-seg shaped wafer LE with distance Rx RE; sample frame glazed to show Sola LVA bifocals, RE 25 mm seg, LE 38 m seg.

The Zeiss LVA range includes a D-segment magnifying bifocal in 1.5×, 2×, 3×, and 4× magnification in which the magnifying segment is cemented onto the support lens. There is no nasal decentration so the spectacles are described as being for monocular use only, with the weaker eye segment frosted. Distance R_x ±10 in highest meridian, cyls to 6DC.

If higher magnification is required the Keeler LVA12 units provide a round segment, 2× to 9× magnification. The bifocal segment is screwed into a trephined afocal or prescription carrier lens or may be fitted into a plastics ring cemented onto the carrier lens. The trephined unit effectively positions the magnifying segment closer to the eye and improves the field of view. On the other hand, if a significant cyl is required in the reading area, the cemented system must be used. The unit can be fitted into any style of frame and gives a wide area of distance vision round the segment with good centration control. The other eye can have a frosted segment if desired. This is an inconspicuous aid with good image quality and the added flexibility of interchangeable magnifying buttons.

(4)   *Clip-on spectacle magnifiers* (Fig. 6.6)

Flip-up, clip-on magnifiers for attaching to a patient's existing spectacles are available in monocular or binocular form.

Power range:
>   Monocular +6.00D, +10.00D, +15.00D
>   Binocular +3.00 to +10.00DS

The binocular units are attached to a bar approx 5½ cm long but the monocular units are virtually in contact with the spectacle lens when in use.

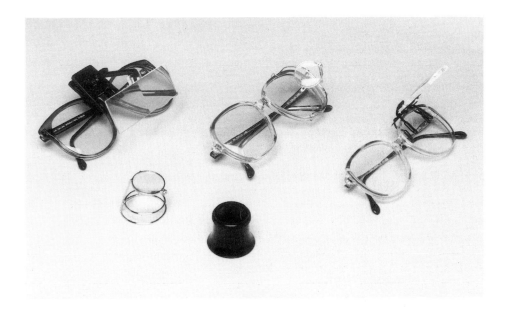

Fig. 6.6 Clip-on spectacle magnifiers and watchmaker's eyeglasses. Eschenbach binocular clip-on magnifier, 4DS to 10DS power; Clip-on watchmaker's eyeglass, 10DS to 20DS power; COIL Magniclip 6DS, 10DS and 15DS power. Also illustrated, conventional watch-maker's eyeglass, power range approximately 10DS to 36DS.

The manufacturer's rating gives a misleading comparison with other spectacle mounted lenses since it reverts to the maximum magnification, $\frac{F}{4} + 1$ basis.

Thus the stated magnification of the clip-on unit only equates directly to a spectacle lens if the equivalent power F_{eq} of the clip-on lens plus spectacle lens combination $(F_1 + F_2 - dF_1F_2)$ is equal to the dioptric power of the single lens spectacle magnifier.

Rayner's Ary hinged, flip-up, clip-on watchmakers' eyeglasses are produced in a range of powers from +10.00D to +20.00D. In theory they can be attached to any frame but in practice it can be difficult to fit them to the modern large eyesize styles.

These clip-on units are lightweight, useful ways of supplementing vision through normal spectacles for specialised more demanding visual tasks.

(5)   Headband magnifiers (Fig. 6.7)

Low power binocular systems attached either to an adjustable headband or spectacle frame. The lens unit is hinged to enable it to be easily tilted into and out of the field of view. Headband units can be used over normal spectacles.

Power range: +2.00D to +10.00D giving a working distance range of 50 cm to 14 cm from the user's face.

Lenses are glass or plastics and incorporate base-in prism. A possible aid when cosmetic appearance is not important, hands need to be left free and a modest power is all that is required.

(6)   Watchmakers' eyeglass-type units (see Fig. 6.6)

Standard watchmakers' eyeglasses are used directly on the face wedged under the eyebrow in front of the orbit.

Power range: +4.00D to +36.00D; stated magnification $\frac{F}{4} + 1$, 2× to 9×.

Lens aperture is in the region of 25 mm, plastics mounting, sometimes with an air hole, glass or plastics lenses. These are of limited use as an LVA but occasionally can be useful for specific small detailed tasks.

6.2   Telescopic units

6.2.1   Optical principles

A near vision telescope or telemicroscope (American terminology) is the magnification device of choice when the patient requires both hands free, but the task necessitates a longer working distance than is available with single lens, microscopic units.

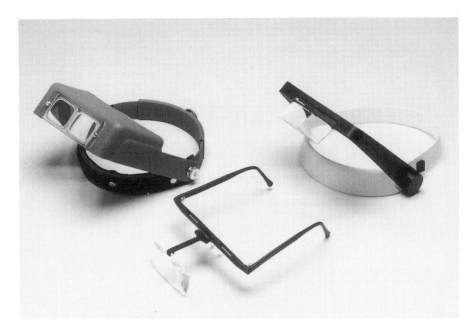

Fig. 6.7 Headband units. Optivisor and Eschenbach headband and spectacle frame option.

The 'balancing act' inherent in the characteristics of aids however, means that the increased working distance of a near vision telescopic unit is gained at the expense of the field of view and depth of field. The three elements are inextricably linked. For any given magnification, a single vision lens has the shortest working distance with the largest field of view, and a slightly more 'forgiving' depth of field (although the object positioning is still quite critical). If a longer working distance is the prime requirement, then the user must accept a reduced field of view and cope with the problems associated with the minimal depth of field. Older patients in particular, with limited accommodation, tend to complain that they 'hardly have to breathe' and they have lost the focus.

Fig. 6.8 is a practical illustration of this field of view/working distance relationship. A comparison is made between four 4× magnification units when used monocularly by normally-sighted, young observers. No attempt is made artificially to control accommodation. The figures given are averages determined experimentally, and would be expected to vary slightly with different observers. As such they do therefore represent the typical performance of such units in use. The figure also highlights some of the user problems associated with such units, namely that even the optimum field of view is small, slowing reading speed, and the 'longer working distance' is still short and in no way resembles a normal reading/close work situation.

As discussed previously, (see section [4.4]) an unmodified distance telescope used for near vision would require massive accommodative effort. It is transformed

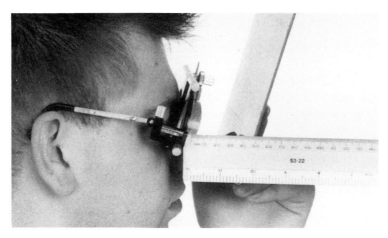

(a)   Unit: Keeler LVA 10. Single vision lens. Effective Ø 30 mm. W/D approximately 6 cm from spectacle plane, 5 cm from front of lens. Average F of V 60 mm, equivalent to 44 N8 size letters.

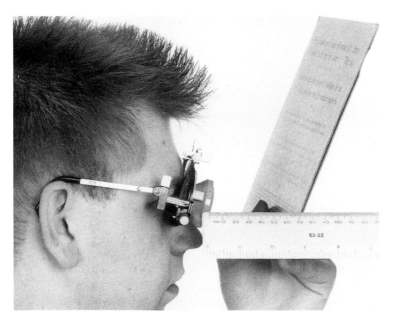

(b)   Unit: Keeler LVA 22. Wide angle telescopic unit. W/D approximately 9 cm from spectacle plane, 7 cm from front of unit. Average F of V 45 mm, equivalent to 34 N8 letters.

Fig. 6.8   Experimental illustration of working distance/field of view relationship. 4× magnification units, one aspheric high plus lens, i.e. microscopic system, and three near vision Galilean telescopic units.

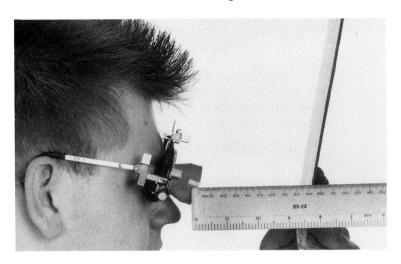

(c)   Unit: Keeler LVA 21. Telescopic unit. W/D approximately 13 cm from spectacle plane, 10 cm from front of lens. Average F of V 30 mm, equivalent to 22 N8 letters.

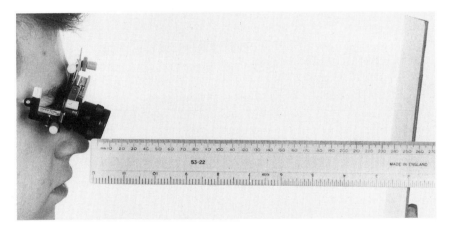

(d)   Unit: Eschenbach 1137/1. Telescopic unit. W/D approximately 30 cm from spectacle plane, 25.5 cm from front of unit. Average F of V 32 mm, equivalent to 23 N8 letters.

into a near unit by the simple expedient of placing a low powered plus lens in front of the objective of the telescope to neutralise the divergent incident light (Fig. 6.9).

As may be seen from the diagram the working distance of the unit is determined by the power of this supplementary lens. A +4.00D lens will give a working distance 25 cm from the front of the objective, a +10.00D lens a working distance 10 cm from the front of the unit and so on. Again, to be technically correct in terms of thick lens theory, one should refer to FVP, rather than simply to the power of the cap.

Since we are dealing with angular magnification, the total magnification of the unit is the *product*, not the *sum* of the nominal magnifications of the two components.

Example:
Basic telescope 3× }
Cap +8.00D (2×) }   Total magnification 6×, WD 12.5 cm.

Basic telescope 2× }
Cap +12.00D (3×) }   Total magnification 6× WD 8.5 cm.

Thus it may readily be seen that the working distance of any given near telescope is determined by the manufacturer's choice with regard to the relative strengths of the basic telescope and the cap. Two equally powerful units may have quite different working distances (Fig. 6.8).

As a generalisation, near vision telescopes based on Galilean principles are more compact, but have a shorter working distance than equivalent power astronomical units. The Galilean system is usually of lower power than its astronomical equivalent, so the supplementary cap has to be more powerful to achieve the same total effect. The higher powered caps inevitably produce shorter working distances.

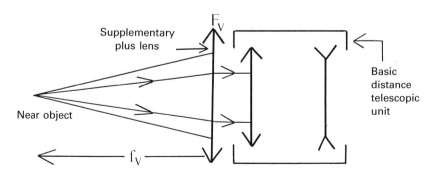

Fig. 6.9 Basic optics of a near vision telescope.

The supplementary power can be achieved either:

(1) By means of a lens cap which the patient attaches to the basic telescope as desired;
(2) By combining the supplementary lens and the objective lens powers to produce a fixed focus unit, or
(3) By varying the separation of the eye piece and objective lens to form a variable focus unit.

Small amounts of spherical ametropia can be neutralised by the patient adjusting the position of the object. An uncorrected myope may hold the object closer than the designated working distance, producing divergent emergent light; uncorrected hypermetropes move things further away, thus increasing the effective working range.

When using focusing telescopes, rather greater amounts of spherical ametropia may be neutralised by adjusting the tube length, i.e. varying the lens separation. When using fixed focus telescopes, significant astigmatism and moderate amounts of spherical ametropia should be corrected in the spectacle carrier lens or in a purpose designed cell behind the eyepiece lens. Uncorrected astigmatism in particular degrades the image quality and may result in the need for a higher level of magnification than would otherwise be the case. Astigmatism in excess of 1.00D should be checked empirically to establish the need for cylinder inclusion in the system.

Telescopes are of fixed focus or variable focus design.

6.2.2   Fixed focus spectacle mounted telescopic units

Almost all are Galilean-based systems.

(1)   *Separate cap designs* (Fig. 6.10)

Rayner 'Telecap', Keeler Multicap telescope (Reference 51), Nikon Near-View attachment range, Bier-Hamblin telescopic units and Zeiss telescopic spectacles are all examples of a low magnification Galilean telescope unit with a supplementary cap which clips or slides onto the objective lens.

Basic telescope magnification is 1.75×, 1.8× or 2×, making up to 2× to 8× total magnification. Most are full aperture lenses although the Zeiss and Bier-Hamblin models are produced as a half lens Franklin-type bifocal. The Keeler Multicap unit features a basic distance telescope to which is fitted a hinged double cap giving the alternative or reading power (2×, 3×, or 4×) or 'TV' lens of 2 m focal length.

All these near vision units are intended for monocular use. The basic telescope

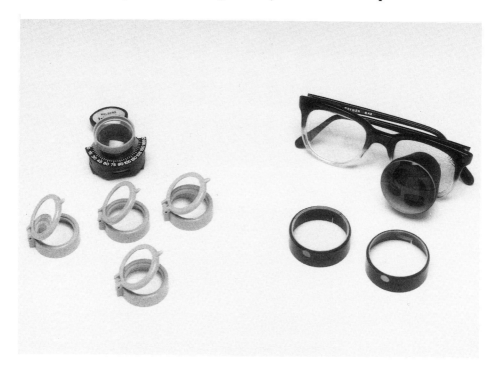

Fig. 6.10 Separate cap, near telescopic units. Keeler Multicap unit (ref. 51), Rayner Telecap glazed for patient use with distance and higher powered supplementary near caps.

may occasionally be dispensed as a binocular distance unit but the weaker eye would have an occluding cap fitted when in use for near vision tasks.

Rayner Telecap and Stigmat units feature the alternative design of a basic near vision telescope with a choice of additional plus power caps to increase the magnification, or a negative power cap to give distance vision magnification. Ametropic correction can be incorporated into the carrier lens for all these units.

(2)   Integral fixed focus systems (Fig. 6.11)

These are units in which the supplementary lens power has been added to that of the objective lens.

Examples of this design are the Keeler series 21 and 22 lenses and the Rayner Telemag design. Nikon main near-view lens, Hamblin high definition units and tiny miniaturised Zeiss 2× magnifying spectacles also come into this category of aid.

Keeler 21 series (magnification 2× to 5×) are unusual in having a standard

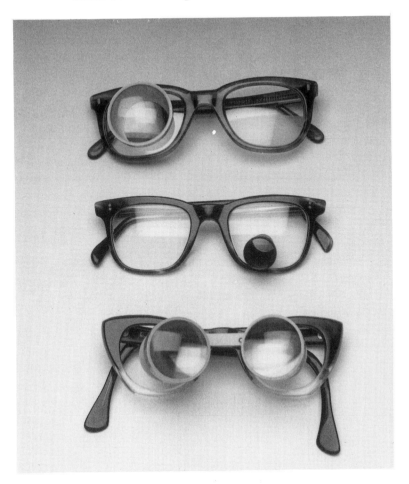

Fig. 6.11 Fixed focus near telescopic units. Keeler LVA 22, RE, LE distance Rx with lower half frosted to minimise confusion from second eye when doing close work; Zeiss 2× magnifying spectacle; Keeler binocular LVA 21 fitted to angled PD bar.

focal length of 16 cm for all lens magnifications. This relatively long working distance enables the units to be prescribed for binocular use, either screwed into plastics PD bars or fitted to angled plastics sleeves cemented directly onto the carrier lenses. It can obviously be used monocularly if prefered.

The series 22 lenses are the 'full-field' version which may be binocular at 1.6×, 2×, and 3× levels but must be monocular above that. Magnification range up to 8×.

The Rayner Telemag has a lightweight black plastics housing and is available as a television viewing unit, or with intermediate 'arm's-length' focus or a choice of five near magnification levels from 1.75× to 8×.

Hamblin High Definition units may be binocular at 2× or 3× magnification but monocular thereafter, 4×, 5×, and 6×.

Zeiss magnifying spectacles differ from these other units in being tiny Galilean telescopes of fixed 2× magnification but available with four different focal lengths from 540 mm to 260 mm. The exceptionally small size of the unit provides extensive distance vision round the unit. Binocularity is easily maintained but the field of view is inevitably very restricted.

Mention should be made of three other units from the Zeiss range, which although extremely expensive, are rather different to the units considered so far. Their prism magnifying spectacles A, C and D are Keplerian (i.e. astronomical) telescopes mounted onto a plastics afocal or prescription lens in a specially reinforced frame.

Spectacle A is a monocular distance telescope with a clip-on lens whose basic magnification, at 3.8×, is twice that of Galilean systems. This enables high levels of near magnification to be provided with a much longer working range. Spectacle C is a binocular version of design A, while spectacle D is a near vision only binocular telescope with an even longer focal length. The magnification range is up to 8× (unit D) and 10× (units A and C), but still at these powers provide the exceptional working distance of 20 cm and 15.5 cm respectively.

The Keplerian system optics also produce a relatively better field than is available through a Galilean system (see Section [4.3.3]), while still retaining the advantage of the longer working distance. The negative side of the equation is the very much greater size, weight and expense of these Keplerian astronomical systems.

Figures derived from Zeiss technical specifications and from the Keeler Manual comparison charts, provide a clear illustration of the relationship between field of view, working distance and unit length for near-vision telescopes and microscopic spectacles (Table 6.1).

Table 6.1 Comparison of working distance, field of view and unit length for various near vision spectacle mounted units.

Comparative figures for 5× magnification units

Unit	WD	FofV	Unit length
Zeiss Galilean telescopic spectacle	13 cm	42 mm	26 mm
Zeiss prism Keplerian spectacle	24½ cm	41 mm	50 mm
Keeler LVA 21 Galilean telescopic	16 cm	25 mm	15–35 mm
Keeler LVA 22 Full-field Galilean spectacle	9½ cm	45 mm	16–22 mm
Keeler LVA 10 wide-angle microscopic spectacle	5 cm	55 mm	minimal
Keeler LVA 12 bifocal microscopic spectacle	5 cm	45 mm	minimal

6.2.3   Variable focus near spectacle mounted telescopic units (Fig. 6.12)

Specifically close range units are few. Eschenbach produce 3× and 4× binocular or monocular clip Galilean design telescopes both designed with a 25 cm working distance. However, since the working distance has been held constant, the single unit increase in magnification halves the field available (see Table 6.2).

Other than these Eschenbach models, units in this category are likely to be extra-short focus roof prism distance monoculars, used in their near-vision mode, with extended tube length. The effective increase in the objective lens power as it is moved away from the eyepiece produces an increase in magnification. The magnification increase with this change from distance to near use, taken from the manufacturer's literature, is given in Table 6.2.

Within each optical system, the field of vision is influenced by the magnification and the diameters of the component lenses. As seen in previous examples, these figures again illustrate the relative field improvement at higher magnification levels associated with the astronomical system optics.

These smaller roof-prism monoculars can be obtained as true spectacle

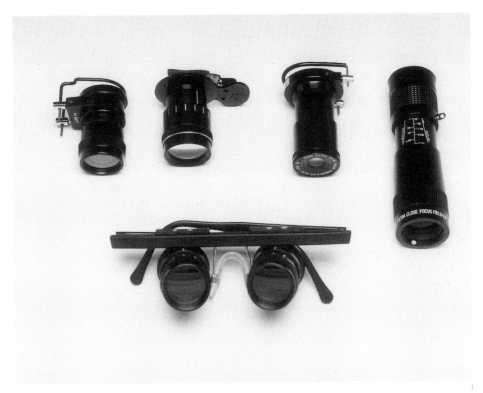

Fig. 6.12 Variable focus near telescopic units. Illustrated: Eschenbach 1137 near telescope (3× or 4×); Keeler Clip telescope in near focus setting; 4 × 12 and 8 × 20 Roof Prism monoculars also in near focus adjustment; Eschenbach 1136 telescopic spectacles (3× or 4×).

Table 6.2 Technical specification, variable focus near telescopes.

Magnification as distance telescope	Near focus	Magnification as near telescope	Field at near focus range
(a) Roof prism astronomical telescopes			
2.75 × 8	15 cm	3.4×	26 mm
4 × 12	20 cm	5×	35 mm
6 × 16	26 cm	7.6×	36 mm
(b) Eschenbach Galilean Units			
N/A	25 cm	3×	70 mm
N/A	25 cm	4×	35 mm

mounted units or fitted to clips to attach to spectacles as required. The larger 8 × 20 units are really too heavy for spectacle attachment. If absolutely desperate however, it is possible to get such a unit made up. Very thick, solid frames are needed and the patient may well need to attach a sport-type securing band to the frame to stop the sheer weight of the telescope dragging the glasses off the nose.

6.2.4   Summary: telescopic systems

The longer working distance associated with near vision telescopic systems renders binocular systems a more feasible option. Binocular units are available up to 5× magnification. The option should, of course, be considered if there is a convincing improvement in visual performance under binocular viewing conditions.

I would, however, suggest that practitioners exercise a degree of caution with respect to the need for binocular units and retain a firm sense of reality when judging improvement in binocular, compared to monocular performance. If the difference is comparatively slight, stick to monocular units. Binocular units are expensive and correct centration and angling is crucial to success.

It is difficult to get the positioning precisely right, but (unfortunately) all too easy to get the setting just slightly wrong, rendering the unit unusable.

Every autumn, new pupils from all over the country arrive at a large boarding school for visually handicapped children in the area in which I work. A full LVA assessment is carried out as soon as they have settled in. It is not uncommon to find they have been provided with binocular telescopic spectacles – but only one unit is still attached to the glasses, the other is languishing in the case! The conversation goes something like: 'the hospital at home arranged for me to have these glasses, but everything was all jumbled up when I looked through both lenses, so I took one off. They are fine now, and I can use my other eye to look around the room and see what's going on. When both lenses were on I had to keep taking the glasses off all the time to see what was happening.'

6.3   Comparative summary of near-vision magnification options

6.3.1   Hand magnifiers

- Comparatively low magnification.
- Light and easy to carrry around.
- Binocular viewing at 'normal' viewing distances.
- May be internally illuminated.
- Inexpensive.
- Require a steady hand.
- Patient must select and maintain focus position.
- May be used with distance or reading spectacles.

6.3.2   Stand magnifiers

- Wide range of magnification available.
- Fairly light weight, but bulky to carry around.
- Binocular viewing possible with lower powers.
- May be internally illuminated.
- Inexpensive.
- Suitable for patients with shaky hands.
- Pre-set focus position.
- Generally require the use of reading spectacles.

6.3.3   Spectacle mounted, non-telescopic magnifiers: microscopic units

- Leaves hands free.
- Comparatively light-weight and inconspicuous.
- Single vision or bifocal units.
- Short working distance.
- Relatively good field of view.
- Illumination can be a problem.
- Usually monocular.
- Medium price range.

6.3.4   Spectacle mounted telescopic units

- Leaves hands free.
- Bulky and conspicuous in use.
- Near use only, obscure distance vision.

- Longer working distance.
- Smaller field of view.
- Critical depth of focus.
- May be binocular up to 5× magnification.
- Expensive.

Questions

1. Compare and contrast the advantages and disadvantages of telescopic and non-telescopic spectacle mounted units.
   (See section [6.1.2].)

2. What would you consider to be the practical upper power limit for a near add being prescribed for binocular use by a patient with equal acuities? How would you decide on the level of base-in prism to relieve the convergence demand?
   (See section [6.1.3].)

3. How is the magnification specified for a 'microscopic' unit – i.e., a high plus lens in the spectacle plane?
   (See section [6.1.1]; [6.1.5].)

4. Many microscopic or near vision telescopic units are supplied for monocular use. What do you do with the other eye?
   (See section [6.1.6].)

5. What are the alternative methods of converting a distance telescope into a near telescope?
   (See section [6.2.1].)

6. What determines the total magnification of a near telescopic unit? What determines the working distance of the near unit?
   (See section [6.2.1].)

7. What magnification levels are available in spectacle mounted form?
   (See section [6.1.6]; [6.2.2]; [6.2.3].)

8. How may you achieve magnification for an intermediate (e.g. arm's length) task?
   (See section [6.2.3].)

9. In what way might a patient's underlying (a) spherical or (b) astigmatic refractive error influence the appliance selection?
(See section [6.2.1].)

10. You are explaining the four basic methods of providing near vision magnification. What are the key points that you would discuss with a patient?
(See section [6.3].)

CHAPTER 7

Individual Patient LVA Assessment, Management and Training

7.1   LVA assessment

By the end of the basic refractive routine, and after discussion with the patient, the practitioner should be in possession of the bulk of the information needed to start to make an intelligent selection of trial aids. An itemised check-list is useful for the less experienced, to help narrow down the large range of possible units.

 (1)   Distance and near VA?
 (2)   Task size?
 (3)   Task working distance and angle of view?
 (4)   Duration and frequency of task?
 (5)   Mix of visual tasks and viewing distances?
 (6)   Any particular visual field or pathology considerations?
 (7)   Does the task require the use of both hands?
 (8)   Steady hands or 'a bit shaky'?
 (9)   Lighting considerations?
(10)   Stable or variable VA?
(11)   Motivation, patient's age and duration of visual disability?
(12)   Financial considerations?

It is helpful to summarise the relevant factors in this way. The experienced can amalgamate and group many of the points together, rapidly mentally rejecting unsuitable aids. The final choice must always be made by the patient, but being presented with a bewildering array of magnifiers and spectacles leads to confusion and is an inefficient use of time. Some pre-selection by the optometrist is essential.

Patients who only want to do a limited amount of reading (their post and occasional 'bits and pieces') are comparatively straightforward to deal with. A single consultation may suffice. Those needing assistance with occupational requirements or aspects of a particular hobby are often more complex. Several sessions may be needed. The first will be devoted to establishing the basic problems and introducing the person to the options and limitations of LVAs. Subsequent visits will improve and refine ideas and solutions as the person becomes more experienced and practiced in the use of various types of aid available.

(1) *Distance and near VA*

This should be established at the end of the routine refraction.

(2) *Task size*

Many normally sighted people only ever open a paper to find out 'what's on TV' so it is a great mistake to assume that all visually impaired people require N5 and are yearning to read *The Times* from start to finish! The key thing is to establish what is required.

I have a vivid memory of a 12 year old partially sighted boy requesting an appointment, his magnifiers were no good anymore, he wanted spectacles instead. I knew he was doing well at school and had rejected spectacle mounted units in the past, so I enquired into the reason for the sudden conversion. He had started studying biology, found it fascinating and wanted his hands free to examine 'things'. Foolishly, I pursued the enquiry: 'What sort of things?' A matchbox was produced from a pocket and I was enthusiastically presented with a large, hairy, decidedly annoyed, spider! An action which precipitated possibly the fastest LVA assessment ever conducted.

Despite such occasional unexpected consequences it is very helpful if the patient brings along examples of the types of object which cause difficulty. Such things as documents, computer printouts, seed catalogues, knitting patterns and so on are comparatively common, but it could equally well be bits of machinery, examples of handicrafts or my young naturalist's spider. In other words, anything the person particularly wants to see.

This is sometimes the only way to be sure about the task detail size, since non-one could possibly be familiar with all hobbies and industrial processes with which patients might potentially be involved.

Knowledge of the VA and task detail required, equated approximately to N-sizes, enable the practitioner to predict the likely magnification which will be needed.

(3) *Working distance and angle of view*

A long working distance requirement is likely to involve telescopic units or hand or stand lenses with a longer focal length, i.e. low magnification units. A stand magnifier may be satisfactory for objects positioned flat on a horizontal surface, but not for objects in a vertical plane which might need a flexible arm unit or a hand lens held in a flexible clamp.

It is sometimes necessary to ask the person to go away and accurately to measure the working distance required before the unit selection can be finalised.

(4)   Duration and frequency of task

Does the person want magnification occasionally to read phone numbers, or all day long on inspection work? Long-term activity needs a higher VA if it is to be resolved in comfort for long periods. For example, a task equivalent to 6/18 size detail would need resolving power equivalent to 6/9 for prolonged viewing.

The duration of the task may also influence the acceptability or otherwise of the field of view of various aids. A very tiny field of view may be tolerable if only needed occasionally for a few minutes at a time, but is likely to be impossibly tiring and frustrating for prolonged use.

(5)   Mix of visual tasks and viewing distances

Is the person concentrating exclusively on a near task or is there a need for a mixture of distance and near vision? If spectacle mounted, will a single vision lens be suitable or would a half-eye, bifocal, or flip-up clip-on design be more appropriate? Is a spectacle mounted unit desirable, or could a hand or stand lens do the job just as well, being picked up and put down as necessary?

(6)   Visual field or pathological considerations

Here one is considering the likely effects of monocular as opposed to binocular units, and wider field non-telescopic compared to telescopic designs.

Patients with nystagmus or patchy, irregular field defects (e.g. some diabetic retinopathies) may achieve better acuity with binocular units if feasible at the magnification level required. Many large, lower powered hand and stand magnifiers retain binocular vision, depending to some extent on the position in which they are held relative to the eyes. Modest magnification requirements (up to approximately 3×) can be achieved binocularly with headband or spectacle clip units and microscopic units incorporating base-in prism. Binocular magnification up to 5× is available with some near vision telescopic units.

Does the patient have a more specific field defect, and if so, where? Is it central (e.g. macular degeneration) or peripheral (e.g. glaucoma or retinitis pigmentosa) or is there more evenly reduced vision but with a full field (e.g. albinism, nystagmus, generalised corneal dystrophy)?

A bifocal construction imposes an additional restriction on the already limited field inherent in all magnification devices. Patients with a significant field loss often achieve better results with a full-aperture unit. For the same reason, elderly patients combining a normal strength reading prescription with a hand or stand lens for occasional use tend to cope better if their spectacles are single vision lenses rather than bifocals. Both types of person benefit from the greater flexibility of head/eye/magnifier/object positioning which is available with full aperture rather than bifocal spectacles.

(7)   Does the task require both hands to be free or not?

If it is essential to have both hands free than a headband or spectacle unit, flexible arm or large stand magnifier will be needed.

(8)   Steady hands or 'a bit shaky'

Any type of device can be considered for someone with steady hands and good manual control. Shaky hands cut down the options considerably, ruling out the use of hand held magnifiers and causing difficulties with spectacle mounted units which have limited depth of focus and require that the object be positioned fairly critically at the correct focal distance.

A stand magnifier or table mounted unit is a much more practical proposition. The choice between the two is going to depend (a) on the power required and (b) on size and requirement for a portable or fixed position unit.

(9)   Lighting considerations

Is there likely to be adequate lighting on the task in the first place?

Does the patient have clear ocular media or are there age/pathological changes to cause significant light scatter or absorption? If so, are the opacities central or peripheral with regard to the visual axis and the pupil?

Thus, is an illuminated aid likely to be of benefit or should the practitioner be endeavouring to improve the intensity or directional efficiency of the external illumination? Does the patient need a chat about the importance of lighting in general? (See Chapter 10.)

(10)   Stable or variable VA

Account should be taken of the stability of the eye condition. Some pathologies, diabetic retinopathy being the most common, are inherently unstable and can give rise to quite large variations in acuity in comparatively short periods of time. One should think in terms of aids which can be readily altered or exchanged. Hand or stand lenses obviously come into the category as do lenses in clip-on mountings. Some Keeler and Nikon units are intended to be used in an interchangeable way. Glazed prescription units in individual fashion frames should be avoided if there is a likelihood of significant visual variation.

(11)   Motivation, patient's age and duration of visual disability

Some attempt must be made to assess the patient's motivation. Many aids, especially those supplied to elderly patients are never used. The person, having evolved a way of life without the need for critical vision, prefers to use friends or relatives as 'eyes' when necessary.

Practise and considerable determination is required to achieve a reasonable level of proficiency in the use of any magnification device. This applies even to basic hand or stand magnifiers. It is more difficult still to 'get to grips' with some of the spectacle mounted telescopic units. For many elderly people requiring only occasional help, it is sensible to aim for the simplest and cheapest appliance which will solve their problem.

Younger people, on the other hand, are more adaptable in their approach and often cope readily with close working distances. Clearer media and greater accommodation provide more flexibility and a better focussing range with microscopic and telescopic units which in turn simplifies their use.

Patients with congenital visual defects are frequently much more positive in their approach to optical aids than is the case with people suffering a visual problem of recent onset. The latter group are considerably more difficult to help since they are inclined to compare any magnification device unfavourably with their previously normal visual abilities, rather than relating it to their present impaired state.

(12)   Financial considerations

In a perfect world the cost of appliances would be irrelevant. Patients would be provided with as many and as varied aids as might possibly be of benefit to them. The fact is of course that patients and eye units have finite resources. The aim of assisting people and alleviating problems has to be tempered by the unpalatable reality of an invariably inadequate LVA budget.

In Great Britain, aids are issued on an extended loan basis through the Hospital Eye Service. An efficient after-care system and some form of labelling on aids are helpful in trying to ensure that at least some units are returned when no longer of use. A large proportion of appliances however, are never seen again.

After consideration of all the facts, the range of aids is likely to have been narrowed down to perhaps four or five alternatives for a given task. The practitioner must then help the patient assess the alternatives, making sure the advantages and limitations of each unit are understood.

You, as the professional, have a responsibility to ensure that the selection of 'short-listed' aids is optically and technically sound and realistic in terms of the factors discussed. The choice must be presented to patients in an unbiased, logical way, but the final decision rests with the patient. Frequently the choice appears surprising. There is no way that the practitioner with 'normal' sight can experience the world as it appears to the person with 'abnormal' sight.

The distortion in one lens form may offset the distortion within a particular eye, whereas another of similar power, but of different lens form, may produce the opposite effect. The unpredictability of the outcome is one of the interesting aspects of LVA work.

7.2   LVA provision and educational considerations

For young children, wherever possible, optical provision should be limited to simple refractive spectacle correction, including bifocals as necessary. Magnifiers and 'gadgets' of all kinds are better avoided until the child has mastered the basic concepts of reading and writing, namely that letters group together to form words and words group together to form sentences.

All magnification devices reduce the field of view and distort spatial/distance relationships to some extent. So although it makes individual letters larger, a magnifier may actively hinder learning if the restricted field prevents the child perceiving the overall pattern of letters and words on the page.

Visually impaired children tend to have poorer hand—eye co-ordination and manual dexterity than their normally sighted counterparts. The mechanics of writing can pose greater problems than normal. Further complicating life with a magnifier should be avoided in the early school years.

If, however, the acuity is so low that some form of magnification appears to be essential right from the start, a stand magnifier is preferable in that it allows room for the teacher to get a finger or pointer underneath, to draw attention to a particular object, word or letter.

Illuminated stand magnifiers should be avoided. Children fiddle with them, run the batteries down and generally wreck the units. Hand held magnifiers and spectacle-mounted aids which require adjustment by the child are also contra-indicated since it is impossible to check if the object is in focus and the unit is actually being used correctly.

The optometrist should be realistic about the detail size needed by young children. Standard early reading books use very large letters which are well within the visual capacity of all but the most massively impaired children. N8 is not encountered until the later stages of junior school. Visually impaired children are much more likely to have co-ordination and scanning difficulties hindering their reading and writing progress, than they are to be held back by an inability to resolve the print detail. Most, after all, have built-in accommodation-based magnifiers! Poor distance vision is less of a problem at this stage since most teaching methods for young children are based on small groups with very little formal blackboard work.

The 1981 Education Act made local education authorities responsible for any child likely to have special educational needs, from the age of 2 years upwards. Some authorities provide home teachers from a much earlier stage even than that specified by the statutory regulations.

Procedures vary, but with parental permission, the LEA may be given full medical and visual details concerning a child.

For effective teaching it is clearly necessary that teachers have an understanding of the child's visual situation. They need some appreciation of the detail size that can be seen, the working distance requirements and any particular colour vision or visual field problems which may exist. Without this type of information it is really rather frightening for a teacher to be confronted by a 'blind' child.

Optometrists may well be appropriate persons to explain, initially to parents and later to school authorities, what the technical labels and numbers actually mean in practical terms. They should also take trouble to ensure that the apparently illogical distance:near abilities of the child are understood.

Schools need advice about when, and if, spectacles should be worn. There is an understandable lay-person's fallacy that people who have 'bad' eyes should wear spectacles! Visually impaired myopic children may well read and write much better without correction. So the advice might well be to allow the child to remove spectacles in the classroom but ensure they were worn elsewhere. This might seem a crazy situation to a teacher not in possession of the facts who, if confronted by a partially sighted child removing their thick glasses in the classroom, is likely to insist that they are worn. Communication is essential since another child might well have opposite requirements.

The close working distance used by these children is often a cause of concern to teachers. They may need reassurance that it is normal and in no way detrimental to the child's sight. Specialized lighting needs may also need explanation. This may consist of supplementary local light for certain tasks, or the opposite, protection from glare in large open-plan glass-walled classrooms.

The overwhelming majority of visually impaired children can cope well within a mainstream infant and junior school environment, provided teachers have been given guidance as to the nature of the visual problem. Coventry Education Authority, which has a team of specialist, peripatetic support teachers, successfully integrates totally blind (NPL) children into local mainstream primary schools. Specialist schooling is rarely considered necessary until secondary transfer, when despite the close proximity of Exhall Grange Special School, many visually impaired youngsters continue in mainstream education. By that stage they are 'adult' as far as LVA provision is concerned with the full range of appliances being provided as and when appropriate.

Active communication and co-operation between all those involved with the child, parents, teachers, optometrist and medical staff will contribute enormously to the management and limitation of the handicap imposed by the child's impaired vision.

7.3 Patient management and training

If at all possible arrangements should be made to review patients after perhaps a month or six weeks 'too see how they are getting on'. This follow-up appointment serves two purposes. It is primarily to find out if the aid is satisfactory. Does it fulfil the purpose for which it was supplied? If not, why not? No matter how careful the initial assessment, the consulting room is not the real world. Ultimately there is no substitute for using the aid at home or work. The initial provision might have been a bit experimental or a compromise between optically conflicting requirements. It is quite common to have to change aids after this trial period.

The other purpose served by the follow-up visit is that it imposes an unspoken pressure on the patient really to make the effort to use the aid. This is possibly more valid in the case of elderly patients, who will hopefully be less likely to go home and simply put the magnifier away in a drawer if they know that they are going to have to go back to the clinic and admit that they haven't tried to use it! On a more serious note, the repeat visit does often show up problems of lighting at home, i.e. that the person could demonstrably read within the clinic setting, but was unable to do so at home (Levitt, 1978; Silver *et al.*, 1978). Reassessment of the strength of the aid combined with repeated demonstration and explanation of the significance of suitable lighting is often beneficial.

Thereafter, appointments are as often as appropriate for individual patients. Many settle onto an annual recheck basis.

For many people provision of an optical aid is sufficient in itself to solve their problems. For other people, other additional non-optical help and training is needed if the optical aids and the person's residual vision is to be used to optimum effect.

7.3.1 Reading stands

Many visually impaired children utilising high levels of accommodation and adults using optical aids have to get very close to the print they are reading. Use of a reading stand can improve comfort and performance by positioning print at a more normal, accessible angle (Fig. 7.1).

Gill (1983) identified over 30 models which were then available in Britain. There are table-top, clamp and free-standing designs. Most have adjustable angles, some are adjustable in height and some can be folded for storage.

Information on stands and overbed tables which can be angled for reading is available from the Disabled Living Foundation and from many of the locally-based charities or social service departments.

Reading stands do not really come within the scope of HES loan arrangements, but in the event of financial difficulty it is possible that help might be available via the social services department disablement provisions. A tray propped at an

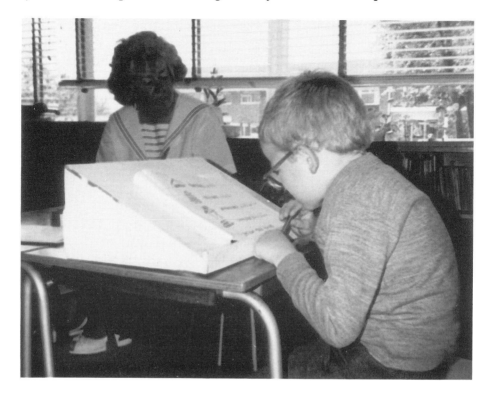

Fig. 7.1 Example of an easily constructed reading stand in use at Exhall Grange School.

angle on a table, or a board across the arms of an armchair supported on cushions, will do as a start. Angled desks for schoolchildren may help comfortable working, in which case responsibility for provision would rest with the education department.

7.3.2   Typoscopes

A typoscope is a matt black plastics sheet or stiff card with a rectangular slit cut in it (Fig. 7.2). Patients may find it valuable to reduce glare and to improve scanning and tracking skills (Backman & Inde, 1979; Collins, 1987).

Many field defects, central, peripheral or hemianopic, cause difficulty when trying to track along a line of print or when needing to locate the beginning of the next line. The typoscope assists the person in tracking accurately along the line and is then slid carefully down to locate the next line.

The matt black surface eliminates reflected glare from the rest of the white paper and may enable the person to increase illumination on the print area uncovered.

The best size of slit will vary with different types of field defect, but may sometimes be estimated from the Amsler chart. For individuals with restricted fields the horizontal length of the slit must be greater than the horizontal dimension of the available visual field. Those with central defects may like a long slit or prefer a narrower one to use one edge as a fixation reference point if reading by eccentric viewing methods.

When used in the normal horizontal position the depth of the slit does not seem to be particularly significant. The patient may keep the slit steady, adjacent to the left-hand margin of the print and move steadily downwards as each line has been completed. It is a matter for personal preference whether the bottom edge of the slit is positioned below the line being read or the top edge positioned above it.

Patients with a very gross field defect may have to move the typoscope horizontally along the line, as well as vertically from one line to the next, in order not to lose their place completely.

Those with a hemianopia may gain benefit from a typoscope used with the slit in a vertical position. Left hemianopias tend to lose the first few letters of each line. Right hemianopias effectively mean that the person is attempting to read 'into' their blind side, a much more severe problem. Positioning the typoscope adjacent to the left-hand side of the column of print gives a much more definite refixation reference point and may be all that the left hemianopia sufferers need to do since they can continue to read with normal scanning movements from left to right. Right hemianopias may need the edge of the print area defined in this way but may also need to employ the steady eye strategy reading principle outlined in the next section.

7.3.3   Eccentric viewing technique – steady eye strategy

These are concepts described by Goodrich & Quillman (1977) and by Backman & Inde in Sweden and now being used with considerable success in England in modified form by the Partially Sighted Society training staff (Collins, 1987).

Macular lesions of various kinds are responsible for a large proportion of the visual problems we encounter. Many of these patients with central field loss discover distance vision eccentric viewing techniques by accident when they find they can see the TV screen, cooker dials and so on, by looking a little away from the object of interest, rather than directly towards it. The preferred direction may be above, below or to either side of the object depending on the size and shape of the scotoma.

It is unusual to find anyone who has spontaneously adapted the idea to near vision tasks without instruction, since the basic eccentric viewing technique (EVT) has to be combined with the so-called, steady eye strategy (SES). It is impossible to utilise eccentric viewing and normal scanning reading movements

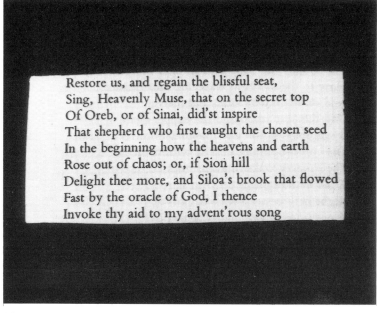

(a)

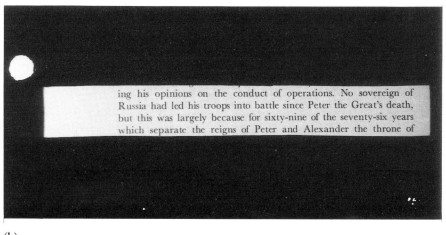

(b)

Fig. 7.2 Typoscope. Examples of various sized slits. An appropriately positioned fixation mark for patients utilising eccentric viewing (b). A large vertical typoscope or strip of card may help locate the start of the line for those with hemianopic defects (c).

at the same time. Anyone attempting to do so will move the image off the preferred retinal area with every eye movement and thus will continually lose their place.

ration and Kutuzov.

Tsar Alexander's views mattered considerably; for, ir
resort, military policy in Russia still depended upon the v
sovereign. It was not until 1802 that a Ministry of War v
in St Petersburg, and even then the military staff continued
themselves as solely responsible to the Tsar himself (a n
concept of loyalty which was only finally broken during
reforms of 1867). Alexander had the ultimate right to dete
disposition of the troops and the direction of strategy. As
Duke he had been trained for military command, most
the Prussianised influence of his father's Gatchina batta
took his soldierly duties so seriously that it was inconcei
would allow his generals to position the army for war witho
ing his opinions on the conduct of operations. No sove
Russia had led his troops into battle since Peter the Great
but this was largely because for sixty-nine of the seventy-
which separate the reigns of Peter and Alexander the t
Russia had been occupied by a woman ruler. The young
not likely to remain in St Petersburg while the rulers of
Prussia and France marched at the head of their regiment

When Russia went to war against France in 1805, Tsar A
set out for Berlin and ultimately for his first campaign, in
He was then twenty-seven years old. So had Napoleon
receiving command of the Army of Italy in 1796; bu
already an experienced veteran. Alexander in 1805 knew
books and all the theory of battle. It was Russia's traged
did not perceive the cruellest schooling was yet to come.

(c)

In normal scanning reading, one keeps the object (i.e. the page) stationary
and moves one's eyes. The steady eye concept requires the patient to identify
the best portion of field, keep the eyes still, and steadily move the print across
this region of the visual field. It is therefore a total reversal of normal habitual
reading procedure. The desire to abandon the eccentric fixation point and look
at the word is very strong at first and it takes a great deal of practice and
encouragement before the SES becomes established.

The first stage is to establish the optimum viewing angle for each person. In
technical terms one is trying to identify the functioning retinal area closest to the
macula, i.e. the area having the greatest potential resolving power.

An Amsler grid is the most convenient device to use. The patient views the grid in good even illumination, ideally wearing full aperture reading glasses. Bifocal lenses may give an artificial result if the person is unable to see the whole of the chart evenly through a small bifocal segment. One can, if necessary, draw out an enlarged Amsler-type grid with black fibre pen on white card.

The person is asked to look towards the centre of the grid. The central spot and surrounding detail will generally be obscured by the central field defect, but common sense and previous experience enable the person to look in the right general direction. While still looking towards the centre of the grid, the person is asked to identify the clearest area of the grid, and then to look in the opposite direction to the clearest area.

As the eye moves, the central spot which was previously missing, generally becomes visible as the functional retinal area is moved into line with the centre of the Amsler chart (Fig. 7.3).

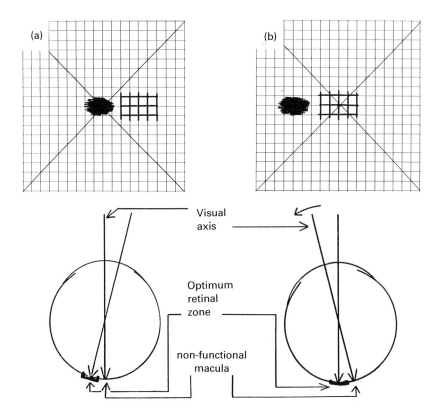

Fig. 7.3 Locating optimum viewing angle in eccentric viewing technique. (a) Preliminary eye position: central scotoma, clearest area to right of fixation. (b) Patient directed to look in opposite direction (i.e. to left) places central spot on functional retina.

The patient will require practice to locate this optimal angle of view. The Partially Sighted Society (PSS), for example, have developed training exercises comprising various sized words surrounded by asterisks which they find are helpful in giving the patient practice in quickly and accurately locating words on the desired eccentric retinal area.

The SES is introduced once this eccentric viewing angle has become 'organised'. Experience is that a patient's reading speed increases rapidly with practice. John Collins, the PSS training officer reports routine increases from 40–60 wpm to 100–150 wpm. It is also found that optical magnification can sometimes be reduced by quite large amounts once this alternative SES has been mastered (Collins, 1987).

A typoscope with an appropriately positioned large white spot on it may sometimes be of assistance in reinforcing the desired angle of view for patients who have difficulty in maintaining the correct steady fixation direction.

It requires a fair degree of practice, and mental and manual organisation but it is possible to combine a stand magnifier with SES reading. The eye-magnifier combination remains stationary, and the print is moved relative to the magnifier, rather than the instinctive action of moving the magnifier along the line of print.

Without doubt the eccentric viewing, steady eye strategy approach can be of enormous benefit to patients with macular area field defects. Unfortunately, although identifying the optimal angle of view does not take long, teaching the person to use the technique is time-consuming.

The ideal approach is a team, incorporating mobility officers, social service or trained voluntary agency staff alongside the LVA clinic optometrists. In the absence of this type of support, as with the use of distance telescopes, limited help and instruction is better than nothing at all.

Normally sighted relatives and friends can play a vital role in the teaching and practice that needs to be done if mastery of SES reading is to be achieved. The 'assistant' should join in and watch the patient getting the basic instruction, working out the optimal viewing angle, and discovering the size of detail that can be resolved. A quick sketch, illustrating the viewing position is very helpful. Also give written instructions reminding of the basic principles of keeping the eye still and moving the print, and of the importance of correct lighting. This is a useful reinforcement, once the person gets home.

A helper is needed in the early stages. Not simply for encouragement, but to assist the person initially to get organised and orientated on the page and to tell them if words are being read correctly and accurate movements made back to the start of the next line. Self-evidently, if you cannot really see what you are trying to read, you cannot be sure if you are right or wrong. An adult struggling to master SES reading techniques is in very much the same situation as a child learning to read for the first time. Both require assistance and someone to provide guidance and correct errors. Struggling along alone is frustrating, dispiriting and unlikely to be successful. Predictably perhaps, the people who experience the greatest difficulty in adapting to EVT and SES are those individuals who were formerly very fast readers. They persist in trying to scan-read with their LVA.

Follow-up appointments are of even greater than normal importance for people trying to master SES techniques. They provide the opportunity to check on progress, to try and sort out problems for those who are struggling, and hopefully to reduce magnification levels for those coping well, thereby potentially improving working distance and field of view. The frequency of appointments is likely to be a compromise between individual patients' needs and the constraints imposed by staff numbers and patient workload.

Successful patients often become demanding patients – in an acceptable sort of way! The solving of one particular problem tends to start patients wondering about assistance for other activities previously given up due to visual problems. There are occasions when the hallmark of success as an LVA practitioner is a patient who arrives with a list of 'things he'd like an aid for' which is longer and more ambitious at follow-up appointments than it was on the initial assessment.

Questions

1   Summarise the factors that you would take into account in compiling a 'shortlist' of aids for a patient.
    (See section [7.1].)

2   How does the duration of the near vision task influence the resolving power/ magnification required?
    (See section [7.1(4)].)

3   What particular factors would you bear in mind when recommending optical aids for a child?
    (See section [7.2].)

4   What aspects of a child's visual performance would a teacher need to know about in order to design a suitable teaching programme?
    (See section [7.2].)

5   What is a typoscope?
    What type of person might benefit from such a device and how might it be used?
    (See section [7.3.2].)

6   Eccentric viewing techniques are of potential benefit to patients with macular problems. How would you establish the optimum viewing angle for such a patient?
(See section [7.3.3].)

7   If utilising eccentric viewing techniques for reading, how must the person modify normal reading methods?
(See section [7.3.3].)

CHAPTER 8
Other Optical Devices

8.1   Field expanders

Restriction of the visual field can impose severe handicap on a person even if the central acuity remains good.

Retinitis pigmentosa is the major pathology involved here although glaucoma and other conditions can, less frequently, give rise to severe field loss with macular sparing.

There have been a number of attempts to develop contact lens-based or spectacle-mounted field expander systems. Such systems are basically either negative lenses or reversed Galilean telescopes. Unfortunately the expanded field is inevitably accompanied by pronounced minification of the image. This reduces central acuity and produces pronounced spatial distortion. Devices have been designed for hand-held occasional use, for mounting in a Halberg clip to use over existing spectacles, or for conventional spectacle-mounted use (Cuifreda, 1977).

Drasdo & Murray (1978) describe a pilot study on the use of visual field expanders on five people with varying severity retinitis pigmentosa. They used spectacle-mounted lens systems and found that despite their severe visual handicaps the patients reacted unfavourably to any device which was cosmetically conspicuous. Of the five people involved in the trial, three rejected the devices totally, either because of cosmetic considerations or because of spatial distortion. The other two subjects did find the expanders of use for some activities at home, but neither made use of them elsewhere.

It is doubtful whether constant use of a spectacle-mounted field expander is a practical proposition. On the other hand, intermittent use of a hand-held, pocketable device, analogous to the way a hand-held magnifying distance telescope is used, might possibly have appeal to a patient.

Devices available are either 'door-spy' systems or large negative lenses such as the Eschenbach 'minifying reader' which is a biconcave, 75 mm diameter glass lens with a 'demagnification' of $-2.5\times$. A basic Galilean telescope of $2\times$ magnification, used as a reversed field-expander unit will produce a halving of the image size with a $4\times$ enlargement of field size (Dowie, 1988).

8.2 Spectacle aids for field defects

8.2.1 Hemianopia mirror systems

Patients suffering from a homonymous hemianopia experience severe mobility and functional difficulties, despite a near normal performance on a letter chart. A mirror attached to the spectacle frame may sometimes be helpful, as a means by which a person may be made aware of large objects/movements, etc., on his or her blind side (Bailey, 1982; Dowie, 1988).

As may be seen from Fig. 8.1 the image of objects reflected in the mirror is superimposed, laterally reversed, on the normal field of view. Head movement causes a very rapid, accelerated movement of the reflected image. The plane mirror is attached to the nasal rim of the frame, before the left eye in cases of left homonymous hemianopia, and before the right eye for right hemianopias.

The size and angle of mounting of the mirror determines the location and extent of the reflected field. However, it will be observed that the mirror inevitably obscures some of the directly viewed field normally available to the

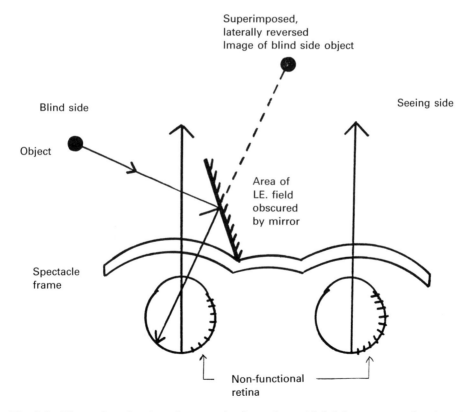

Fig. 8.1 Plane mirror hemianopia spectacles for patient with left homonymous hemianopia.

eye behind the mirror. A compromise mirror size, 20–40 mm width, is generally used.

The superimposed, reversed image obviously initially causes some considerable confusion for the individual. The users must develop an ability to ignore the image to some extent, while nonetheless using it as a means of becoming aware of significant activity or objects on the blind side. Once aware of the object, the head is turned to examine it directly.

A semisilvered or dichroic mirror is sometimes felt to have advantages over a conventional mirror. The semisilvered principle eliminates the problem of the mirror obscuring a major part of the 'seeing half' of the relevant eye. Instead, the person retains a normal field of view, of reduced intensity, through the mirror, associated with similarly reduced intensity, reflected images from the blind side (Fig. 8.2).

The dichroic mirror transmits blue light and reflects red light. The user therefore experiences red reversed images superimposed on a blue-tinged normal half field. It is claimed that the semisilvered principle preserves a more normal, comfortable stereoscopic vision on the seeing side. Introducing the coloured

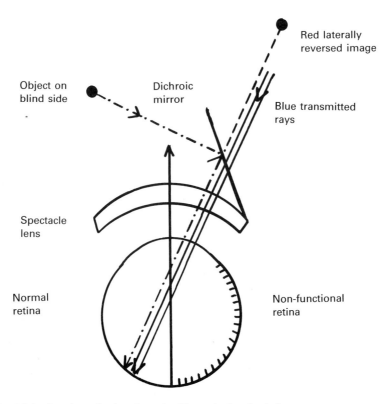

Fig. 8.2 Dichroic mirror for hemianopia. Example for the left eye.

images may then further assist the person to differentiate the real from the reflected view.

Most patients find the mirror system disorientating and difficult to manage so the success rate is inevitably low. Nevertheless, hemianopia sufferers do have a particular problem which can sometimes be helped in this way. Dichroic mirrors are available from Rayner Optical Co, either fitted and hinged to a metal spectacle frame, or hinged to a Halberg test clip for trial purposes. If this ready-made unit is not suitable, wire, solder, glue and ingenuity will be required on the part of the practitioner!

8.2.2 Prism based systems

The severe mobility and orientation problems experienced by hemianopia sufferers are shared by anyone with a severe field restriction. Advanced glaucoma and retinitis pigmentosa are obvious examples of the types of pathology involved.

An excellent review of the principles underlying the use of prisms for such patients is given by Bailey (1978). He states that 'the purpose of the prisms is to create a displacement of the peripheral field on the "blind" side, shifting it towards the primary visual direction. This has the effect of reducing the magnitude of the eye movement necessary for looking at, or searching for, objects on that "blind" side'. Small segments of Fresnel prism are attached to the spectacle lenses with the prism base in the same direction as the field restriction.

The person starts by viewing through the normal spectacle lens, makes a gradual eye movement towards the blind area, reaches the prism, experiences an image jump, and then views through the prism. The scale of the scanning eye movement will depend on the positioning of the edge of the prism. The power of the prism determines both the magnitude of the jump and the relative decrease in the eye movement required for viewing objects in that region of the visual field. There will also be a monocular scotoma at the edge of the prism whose extent corresponds to the prism power (Fig. 8.3).

The size, position and power of the Fresnel segment will obviously depend on the nature of the field defect. Assuming a spectacle plane to centre of rotation distance of 27 mm, Bailey gives a rule of thumb that every 1 mm movement of the prism edge from the primary position corresponds to a 2° eye rotation. Hence, a prism positioned 5 mm from the pupil centre will not be encountered until the eye turns through 10°.

The majority of patients for whom this type of prism system might be appropriate are likely to have similar field defects in both eyes. Prism segments will be required on both lenses. The substantial powers involved inevitably result in regions in which normal fusion and binocular vision are impossible. In addition to the prism-induced scotomas, there will be regions of diplopia and confusion when dissimilar images are superimposed.

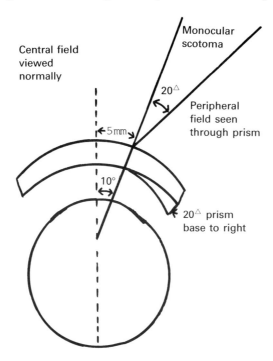

Fig. 8.3 Prismatic management of field defects. A 20^Δ prism placed 5 mm from the centre of the pupil. The monocular scotoma is 20^Δ (11°). The field 38^Δ (21°) or more to the right will be viewed through the prism and will appear displaced inward by 20^Δ (11°). (*After* Bailey, 1978.)

An individual has only a limited range of comfortable eye movements. Beyond that range, scanning requires either undue effort or head movement. The concept underlying the provision of prism for a person with a severe field restriction is to widen the area which can be encompassed within the comfortable scanning range.

Bailey recommends that prisms be considered for all patients with hemianopias or fields that do not extend beyond 10° from fixation. He prefers the prescribing principle of Weiss (1972), suggesting a 15^Δ prism, positioned $3\frac{1}{2}$ mm from the pupil centre for hemianopia patients. Those with concentric field defects are given two prisms on each lens, nasally and temporally, positioned 6 mm from the pupil centre for binocular fields of approximately 10° extent.

Bailey stresses however, that the patient will require considerable counselling, explanation and training in order to understand the purpose and effect of the prism.

8.3   Contact lenses

Certain categories of patient achieve an enlarged, or better quality retinal image when supplied with contact lenses rather than spectacles. Such patients may qualify for contact lens supply through the NHS.

8.3.1   High myopia

Contact lenses give rise to a much larger retinal image and improved field compared to the equivalent power spectacle lens.

8.3.2   Keratoconus, corneal scaring, keratoplasty

Any distortion or irregularity of corneal structure has serious implications for vision if it encroaches into the pupillary area.

Transparent, but uneven corneas, e.g. keratoconus, high post-operative astigmatism, corneal grafts may achieve an excellent standard of vision through a contact lens. The lens fitting can be technically quite difficult, but often results in spectacular improvements in acuity and image quality.

A contact lens cannot eliminate the effect of actual corneal opacity. The position, size and density of the opacity will always be the limiting factor with regard to final acuity. However, scarred or opaque areas (especially if of traumatic origin) are frequently surrounded by zones of clear, irregular tissue. In such eyes a worthwhile improvement in acuity may result from the provision of a contact lens even if the vision is still subnormal. A partially occluding 'pinhole' optic zone might also be worth considering.

From an optical standpoint the majority of such corneal problems are best tackled with a rigid lens material of corneal or scleral design. Soft lenses do have a role however, although corneal vascularisation is inclined to be a perceptibly greater problem than normal.

In cases of high post-operative astigmatism spectacle lenses, although providing 6/6 acuity, may give rise to intolerable levels of meridional spatial distortion or aniseikonia. If there are insurmountable fitting problems, or the person is unable to tolerate rigid lenses, it may be possible to incorporate part of the refractive correction into a soft lens. The residual error would then be corrected by a much reduced strength spectacle lens, thus reducing the spatial distortion or aniseikonia to tolerable levels.

8.3.3   Nystagmus

Many, but not all patients with nystagmus achieve a better standard of vision when corrected with contact lenses rather than spectacles (Abadi, 1979). Nystagmus is frequently associated with a moderately high astigmatic refractive error. When this is the case it is reasonable to suppose that the greater stability of the retinal image associated with contact lens correction will result in improved resolution. However, an improved acuity sometimes results from fitting contact lenses to emmetropic nystagmus patients. It is not clear why this should be so. It seems unlikely that the very slight mass of a corneal or soft lens would damp down the amplitude of the nystagmus to any significant extent.

Clinical experience is also that some patients, even those with quite large refractive errors, do not show any improvement in acuity with a contact lens. It is necessary to assess each patient individually, since it is not possible to predict who will achieve a worthwhile visual improvement. In many instances nystagmus is associated with pathology or abnormality elsewhere in the eye or visual pathways. Even cases of so-called simple congenital idiopathic nystagmus are likely to have a degree of stimulus deprivation amblyopia so it would be quite unrealistic to expect to improve acuity to normal, simply by the provision of a contact lens. Successful contact lens wear requires a fairly high level of patient motivation, such that only the patient can judge whether the improvement in vision constitutes sufficient motivation to render lens wear beneficial. Improvement from 6/12 to 6/9 is of great significance to someone keen to drive, but may pass unnoticed by other patients.

8.3.4　Contact lens telescope

In theory one can provide magnification by constructing a Galilean telescope by means of a high minus contact lens and a high plus spectacle lens. I have attempted this on a number of patients – with a complete lack of success! The difficulty lies in the very high powers required since the separation between lenses is constrained by the practical problem of fitting the spectacles on the nose!

The idea was first suggested by Dallos (1936). Mandell (1965) makes a number of references to such systems, while Bier (1970) states that, 'it is a sound practical proposition where a magnification of 1.6× or less suffices'. Suggestions originally were that scleral lenses should be used to ensure lens stability (Bier & Lowther, 1977), but hydrogels have also been recommended (Stone & Breakspear, 1977).

Despite the very positive sounding literature, Silver & Woodward (1978) document one of the very few examples of a contact lens telescope system actually being used successfully in practice. An improvement in acuity from 6/18+ to 6/9 enabled the patient concerned to pass his driving test. Silver & Woodward stress that the patient must be exceptionally well motivated with a specific problem which will not yield to alternative solutions. The stability of the contact lens is of paramount importance. It is advantageous if the person is hypermetropic or aphakic to increase the potential negative 'eyepiece' power (i.e. eye plus CL), and if they have deep-set eyes to increase the separation of the lens elements. It also helps if the person is already an established lens wearer.

On balance therefore, a contact lens telescope is of more theoretical interest than it is a practical proposition.

8.4 Tints

8.4.1 Tinted contact lens

(1)   Albino babies
Many contact lens practitioners have fitted albino babies with scleral, or more recently, hydrogel cosmetic lenses with a clear pupil and opaque black lining.

It was felt that the multidirectional light entering the eye through the iris as well as through the pupil, retarded the organisation of retinal receptors within the macular area.

The newborn retinal receptor cells were believed to be rather randomly positioned, and that normal organisation and positioning occurred in response to directional light from the pupil, i.e. like plants growing towards the light. It was logical to try and fit an opaque lens with a reduced pupil diameter very early in life in the hope that this would improve cone organisation within the macular area, thus enhancing potential resolution and acuity. The reduced pupil and bulk of the lenses was also felt to reduce the amplitude of the nystagmus, thus again potentially improving acuity.

More recent work however, has shown that macular hypoplasia and absence of macular luteal pigment are the most significant factors contributing to the reduction of acuity in albinism (Fonda, 1962; Mann, 1957). Ruben (1967) considers there is no evidence that contact lenses with reduced pupils can improve vision.

Some albino children are very photophobic. This can be a very difficult management problem if the entire family are not to be consigned to a mesopic existence behind closed curtains! Tinted contact lenses may be the best way of alleviating the photophobia. The child's functional vision will be improved even though the actual VA is unchanged, and the rest of the family will have a much more comfortable life as well. Lenses are generally well tolerated by babies and small children. Refitting is necessary as the child grows, and a close check must be kept on the power. Tinted spectacles should obviously be considered if there are refractive (i.e. high astigmatism) or management problems with soft lenses.

(2)   X-CHROM lens
Red-dyed PMMA lenses were reported by Zeltzer (1971) to 'provide enhanced colour perception in colour defective individuals'. The X-CHROM lens is fitted to the non-dominant eye, with a normal lens fitted if necessary to the dominant eye. Cantor & Silver Ltd have exclusive manufacturing and distribution rights for Britain and Europe. The tint transmission curve shows maximum transmission

in 575–750 nm (orange–red) range with some additional transmission in the 370–480 nm (blue) range (La Bissoniere 1974).

Studies investigating Zeltzer's claims have come to widely differing conclusions Taylor (1984). Some feel the lens has little effect, Siegel (1981) and La Bissoniere (1974) while others concluded the lens was of value (Eger, 1974; Ditmars & Keener, 1976). The lens works best for protanomalous trichromats, although there are reports of successes with deutans and dichromats (Fletcher & Voke, 1985).

The green part of the spectrum is reduced in brightness by the filter, relative to the red part. Subjectively, some colour defective individuals feel their range of colours is improved and that they can distinguish colours more easily while wearing an X-CHROM lens. Objective assessment gives widely varying results, both between individuals and between alternative colour vision assessment systems.

It is important to realise that the lens is merely a possible aid to improve colour perception, not a cure for colour-blindness.

8.4.2   Tinted spectacle lenses

Age related changes in the eye induce a decline in visual function. The effects relate primarily to the pupil, lens and retinal receptors and pigment epithelium.

Ageing effects in the lens are discussed in Chapter 10. Within the retina, there is evidence of a net loss of cones over the age of 40 years (Gartner & Henkind, 1981) with particular loss within the foveal area (Marshall, 1985). Cone outer segment discs are joined together and have a slow replacement rate such that the entire outer segment is renewed only every 9–12 months (Foulds, 1980). On the other hand, rod outer segments are composed of some 1000 discrete discs (stacked like a pile of coins) which have a very rapid replacement rate. Each day 30–100 new discs are made and the entire rod light-sensitive outer segment is renewed every two weeks (Marshall, 1977). Old discs are removed by the phagocytic action of the pigment epithelium. Once within the pigment epithelial cells the engulfed discs are broken down and partially recycled through Brüch's membrane into the choroidal circulation. The number and activity of the pigment epithelial cells declines throughout life such that there is a steady accumulation of incompletely degraded particles within the pigment layer. This accumulated debris tends to displace the overlying pigment cells and becomes visible as the excrescences on Brüch's membrane known as Drusen (Sarks, 1976).

This build up of waste material within the pigment epithelium/Brüch's membrane system is established as a causative factor in senile macular degeneration; it may also be implicated in the various types of pigmentary retinal degeneration.

The advent of lasers and generally stronger, more intense light sources has stimulated research into the varying effects of light on animal and human retinas. Much is still unclear, but damage seems to be sustained both by the photoreceptor cells themselves and by the pigment epithelium. Precise effects appear to depend on the nature, intensity and duration of the incident light. In general terms, however, it seems clear that prolonged exposure to high levels of light is detrimental, particularly to older eyes, and that short wavelength blue light, is of particular concern (Marshall, 1985).

These research results have given rise to the suggestion that protecting eyes from light might retard the deterioration rate in pigmentary degenerative conditions (Adrian *et al.*, 1977; Noell *et al.*, 1966). Research results and clinical trials are now broadly in agreement that filters should absorb short wavelength blue light; they will thus have a red–brown tint (Everson & Schmidt, 1976; Taylor, 1979).

People suffering from retinitis pigmentosa often suffer severe visual problems in bright light as well as the more commonly mentioned night blindness. There are also difficulties associated with sudden changes of light level. This is a result of the abnormally slow recovery rate of the retinal photopigments.

Trials with Corning 550 red photochromic lenses and fixed tint red and brown lenses show a strong preference by RP sufferers for some form of tint. Although some patients evinced a definite subjective liking for one or other tint, there is no evidence that a photochromic tint has any marked advantage over a fixed tint (Silver & Lyness, 1985).

Corning CPS standard photochromic lens range (available from Keeler Ltd) comprises the yellow–orange coloured CPS511 (LTF 47% to 12%), CPS527 (LTF 34% to 9%) which is a stronger orange colour, and the CPS550 red lens (LTF 20% to 5%). The CPS511 and CPS527 are also produced in a slightly darker multilayer coated form. Similar absorption principles apply to the Norville Group PLS range of solid plastics tints. The PLS530 (yellow), PLS540 (orange) and PLS550 (orange-red) tints provide a slightly cheaper fixed tint alternative to the Corning photochromic range.

The strong colour of the red lenses is a cosmetic drawback to some patients – the spectacles do look rather startling – and the inevitable colour distortion is sometimes unacceptable. Both these problems are overcome to a large extent by the Rodenstock Perfalit Lambda 660 block filter tint whose cosmetic appearance is of a golden-brown sunglass lens. The spectral transmission curve of this lens shows a block below 500 nm, limited transmission in the green–yellow range building up to a high transmission above 700 nm. The tint may be applied to any Rodenstock lens and is available in a choice of 80% or 90% absorption (Fig. 8.4).

It is a lens I have found very useful, sometimes with tinted sideshields, for patients with retinal dystrophy, diabetic retinopathy, media opacity or severe corneal dystrophy. A word of warning must however be given to patients with gas appliances. The almost complete block of short wavelength transmission

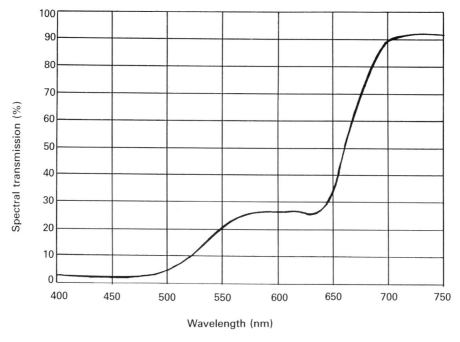

Fig. 8.4   Spectral transmission of Rodenstock Perfalit Lamdba 660 block filter lens. (*Courtesy of Rodenstock UK Ltd.*)

renders a gas flame completely invisible — great care is needed if using gas cookers or lighting gas fires.

Patients with cone dystrophies should always be provided with tinted spectacles. Some are comfortable with conventional photochromic or 30–40% transmission fixed tints but it may be beneficial to give an extremely dark tint, possibly as dense as 2% transmission (Faye, 1984; Silver, 1988).

8.4.3   Amber tints

Light scatter, associated with age-related lens sclerosis and/or early cataract, can be a major cause of discomfort or even disability glare. Short wavelength, blue light is scattered more than longer wavelength light. Amber filters may be beneficial in reducing glare and increasing visual comfort and efficiency both for distance and near vision.

8.4.4   Inherited colour defects

People suffering from inherited colour defects may sometimes be helped by tinted lenses. Fletcher & Voke (1985) recommend the use of a range of magenta (purple—red), red, orange and purple filters of different densities. Performance with the various filters is assessed with pseudoisochromatic tests, after which patients should ideally be loaned filters for a trial period.

Any such filter will selectively alter brightness, hue and saturation of objects, in line with the transmission characteristics of the filter. Ideally, one needs to know the transmission curves of the assessment filters used. However, if using the well-documented Kodak Wratten filters as samples, one may find that it is not possible to accurately reproduce the LTF and transmission curve in dip-dyed plastics prescription lenses.

Patients may also express disquiet at the cosmetic appearance of such tints. Clip-ons may then be an answer to both these difficulties, to be used as required by the patient.

Results are subject to considerable individual variation, but the general pattern appears to be that protan-group defects respond most favourably to red tints, while deutan-type problems find magenta filters most beneficial.

Fletcher & Voke feel that 'if correctly applied, coupled with cautious advice against over-confidence, and stressing the dangers of tiredness and adverse conditions, filters can be prescribed to assist in many cases'.

Questions

1 Field defects can impose a severe handicap on a person even if the central acuity remains good. If attempting to help a person with a right homonymous hemianopia, where on the frame would the mirror be attached? What are the advantages claimed for a dichroic mirror compared to a normal plane mirror? (See section [8.2].)

2 What is the rationale behind the suggested use of peripheral prism for patients with severe concentric field restriction? (See section [8.2.2].)

3 When might a contact lens be considered to be a low visual aid? (See section [8.3].)

4 Discuss the management of total albinism. (See section [8.4.1(1)].)

5 Discuss the use of tinted spectacle lenses for visually impaired patients. What type of ocular problem would be likely to benefit from tinted lenses? How would you decide upon the colour and density of tint? (See section [8.4.2].)

CHAPTER 9

Electronic Aids

9.1   Closed circuit television systems (CCTV)

The first description of the use of a CCTV system as a subnormal vision aid occurs in a paper by Potts *et al.* 1959. Work by Grenensky and colleagues at the Rand Corporation in Santa Monica, California, in the late 1960s and early 1970s was then mainly responsible for establishing the CCTV as an accepted low vision aid (Grenensky, 1969; Grenensky *et al.* 1972).

   Field trials with various prototypes continued throughout the 1970s, both in America and at Moorfields Eye Hospital in London (Silver & Fass, 1977; Silver & Gill, 1979).

   Currently there are some 30 models available in Britain, varying in price from around £1200 to £2100 for black and white models and in the region of £1800 to £2200 for colour models. Full technical specifications are readily available from the manufacturers (see Appendix 5 for addresses). This is a rapidly developing technology with frequent improvements in components and design.

   Excessively detailed comparative descriptions of individual CCTV models are inappropriate here, and would inevitably soon become outdated. However, general characteristics and requirements have been arrived at largely as a result of clinical trials and user experiences, so are likely to remain valid.

9.1.1   Comparison of CCTV systems with optical aids

Advantages

Greater magnification: 3× to 80× depending on monitor screen size.
Variable magnification with zoom lenses.
Relatively normal working distance and reading position.
Reversed polarity: option of white-on-black or black-on-white symbols.
Enhanced contrast.

Disadvantages

Bulky and difficult or impossible to move around.
Expensive.
May require skilled installation and maintainance.

The main variables between currently available models are:

- Black and white or colour.
- Size of monitor screen, from 12″ to 20″.
- Magnification range.
- Manual or automatic focus.
- Intensity and position of illumination.
- Height, adjustment and tilting facility of monitor.
- Availability of underlining and 'windowing' (i.e. typoscope effect).
- Range of brightness and contrast controls.
- Size and movement range of platform.
- Option of black, white, green or amber screen background.
- Split screen/dual camera option.
- Camera position and range of movement.
- Compatibility with computer, typewriter or other electronic equipment.

These last variables affect the flexibility of the unit. Some designs feature a vertical arrangement of an integral monitor/camera unit positioned directly above the platform (Fig. 9.1). This is the most compact arrangement but limits examination of bulky 3D objects. The alternative of a separately mounted camera unit at the side of the monitor allows the possibility of tilting the camera as well as adjusting its vertical position relative to the platform. In some instances the camera can be tilted to a horizontal position. With appropriate lenses it can be used to focus objects at various distances up to infinity (e.g. LVA Ltd MKIV unit or distance camera option).

Flexibility and applications of the CCTV principle are being extended continually. Some models incorporate a split-screen and/or dual camera option. One can, for example, read and see what one is writing at the same time; feed in pictures of two different texts or objects on to the two halves of the screen; input a computer/VDU on to one half while simultaneously viewing conventional printed documents on the other half screen (Fig. 9.2).

Some systems can be adjusted for use with a typewriter. A magnified view of the carriage enables the typist to check the accuracy of the work as it is being done. Models can be linked into composite systems with computers and microfiche units to give a much enlarged print display, or with 'braillers' and with voice synthesiser machines (Figs 9.3 and 9.4).

The reversed polarity option is particularly valuable. An informal survey among children at Exhall Grange School a few years ago found that approximately two thirds of pupils regularly using CCTVs expressed a strong preference for the white-on-black reversed polarity mode. It reduced glare problems and was subjectively more comfortable for prolonged use. In many instances reading speed was improved by changing to the white-on-black setting. Sometimes less magnification was required. Studies of adult CCTV users also commonly show this strong preference for the reversed polarity display. Silver & Gill, 1979; Fletcher, 1979).

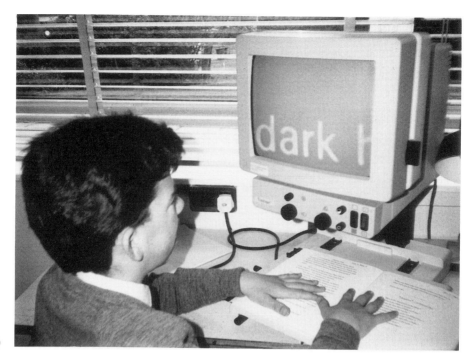

(a)

(b)

Fig. 9.1 Two Vantage CCTV in-line units in classroom use, both set in reversed polarity mode, but showing very different levels of magnification and contrast. (Sensory Visionaid Unit.)

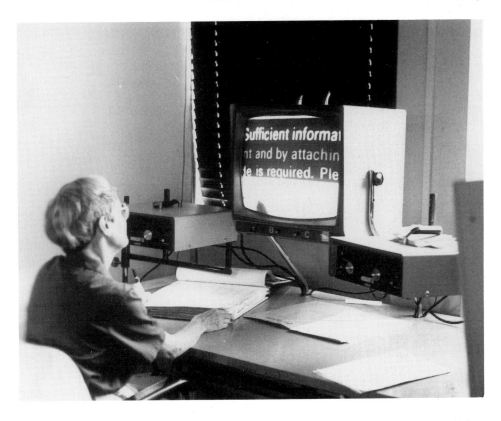

Fig. 9.2 Voyager XL CCTV double camera system. Split screen system, reversed polarity. Information documents are placed under the right-hand camera, left-handed user writes in ledgers placed under left camera. The platforms have been removed from below the cameras to allow thick ledgers to fit more easily underneath. (*Courtesy Coventry City Council Rating Department.*)

Manufacturers are usually very helpful. Anyone considering purchasing a CCTV system should contact the various suppliers individually to establish exactly what variations, permutations and options are feasible within each basic design.

In Britain a number of CCTV systems are purchased privately, although the majority are provided by education departments or by the Training Agency (formerly the Manpower Services Commission).

If required as an aid to employment, CCTV units are funded by the Training Agency who are empowered to provide any type of appliance deemed 'essential to employment' to enable a handicapped person obtain or retain a job.

The initial visual assessment of a prospective CCTV user is done at one of a number of designated hospital-based LVA clinics. Recommendations are passed to the RNIB Employment Services Department. The RNIB, in conjunction

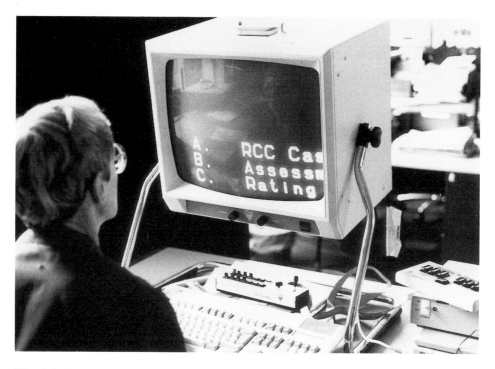

Fig. 9.3 DP11 computer enlargement system. (*Photograph courtesy Coventry City Council Rating Department.*)

with the local BPRO or Blind Persons' Training Officer deal with the person's employer and assess the practicalities of installing the unit at the patient's place of work.

Within schools and colleges for the visually handicapped CCTV use is increasing steadily as a valuable additional option to supplement conventional optical aids. The non-portable nature of the CCTV does nevertheless restrict us value and appeal. You cannot, for example, read in bed or do your homework on the bus with a CCTV!

9.2 Other electronic aids

The electronic microchip revolution is having a beneficial effect on equipment and aids available to braille users and others without useable residual vision. Although, strictly speaking, outside the scope of this book, an awareness of developments in this field will be of interest.

Speech systems (with or without earphones) and braille conversion programmes can be interfaced with some computers and word processor systems. One can obtain talking watches, calculators and brailler machines as well as the Kurzweil

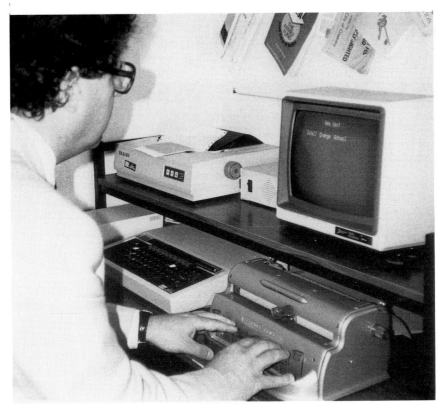

Fig. 9.4 Composite system comprising BBC computer/word processor, printer and screen with optional symbol magnification; Perkins brailler and printer and voice synthesiser. System devised to suit the needs of Richard Bignall, the blind headmaster of Exhall Grange School, Coventry.

reading machines which have been installed in some of the larger public libraries.

Portable hand-held camera systems are expanding the scope and flexibility of electronic systems. The Viewscan unit converts print to a visual display; the Optacon II converts print, graphic images and computer output into a tactile 'image' of vibrating rods sensed by the user's index finger. The Alphavision 'Delta' is a similar portable camera unit which will translate print into a braille tactile display or an optional voice synthesiser.

All innovations are bound to be expensive if manufacturers are to recoup development costs. Nevertheless, the outlook for grossly visually disabled people is more encouraging than ever before. Developments are still at an early stage, but there is a huge potential for improving means of communication and participation by non-visual methods thus enabling blind people to become involved in work and activities previously closed to them.

Questions.

1. In Britain what are the main channels through which CCTVs are provided? (See section [9.1].)

2. Who carries out the assessment of a prospective CCTV user? (See section [9.1].)

3. What levels of magnification are available with CCTV systems? (See section [9.1].)

4. What is reversed polarity? In what way may it benefit a CCTV user? (See section [9.1].)

5. Outline some of the other variables in CCTV design. (See Section [9.1].)

6. Do you know of any other electronic aids which might be of assistance to a blind person? (See section [9.2].)

CHAPTER 10
Lighting, Colour and Contrast

10.1 Lighting

10.1.1 Introduction

The information in this chapter is primarily intended to help those advising patients on ways of improving the lighting within their own homes. Illumination levels in public buildings, offices, factories, schools, etc., are governed by legislation and conform in general to recommendations in the CIBS Code for Interior Lighting, 1984.

It has been known for many years that the normal ageing processes within the eye effectively reduce the amount of light reaching the retina. Weale in *The Ageing Eye* (1963), states that there is in the order of a threefold drop in transmission between a 60 year old compared to a 20 year old eye. Thus when exposed to the same test conditions, an average 60 year old retina receives only one third as much light as is received by the 20 year old retina.

Among the normally-sighted population, visual acuity improves as illuminance increases (Weston, 1961; Boyce, 1978; Julian, 1984). This relationship holds good for many, although not all, visually impaired people.

The two elements of age and illumination are well illustrated in Fig. 10.1, taken from Boyce (1978). The difference in performance in the same proof-reading task is shown related to increasing levels of illumination for young and elderly age groups. It can be seen that although both young and old gain by increasing illumination, the older age group's gains are of far greater magnitude.

Measurement of performance must involve both the quality and the quantity or speed of 'throughput' of the activity. Perception and vision as a whole is far more complex than merely recording visual acuity even for a so-called 'normally sighted' person. The human eye has an impressive capacity to adapt and 'see' over a huge intensity range from 0.1 lux (starlight) up to approximately 80 000 lux (bright sunlight). It would be naive to expect that increasing illumination alone would solve all problems. Nevertheless, intelligent use of lighting, colour and contrast are key contributions to the task of creating an environment in which the visually impaired person is able to make optimum use of vision.

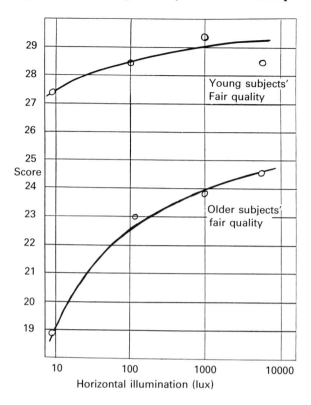

Fig. 10.1 Mimeo Proofreading Experiment. Adapted from P.R. Boyce (1978), 'The Relationship Between the Performance of Visual Tasks and the Lighting Conditions', *Light for Low Vision Symposium.*

Ultimately, as in much LVA work, the patient will be the final arbiter. Certain guidelines are nonetheless helpful.

The optometrist should be aware of potential problems with glare as light source intensities are increased. Lighting experts subdivide glare into two categories, namely:

(1) Discomfort glare: annoying and tiring but producing no measurable drop in VA.
(2) Disability glare: prevents one seeing (i.e. reduces acuity) in the neighbourhood of the glare source.

Some acquaintance with basic lighting terminology is very helpful and a distinction must be drawn between general lighting and specific task lighting. Lighting definitions are listed in Appendix 4.

10.1.2 General lighting

The CIBS/IES Codes give recommended illuminance levels for a huge range of activities. The Code covers industrial and office premises, public buildings, hospitals, etc., but also includes quite detailed reference to homes. The recommendations cover general living areas, stairs, corridors, kitchen work surfaces as well as casual and detailed reading/near vision activity areas.

The code also states quite specifically that illuminance levels should be increased by 50–100% for homes occupied by elderly people (Fig. 10.2).

Studies by Levitt (1978) and Silver *et al.* (1978), although small scale, do suggest that a large proportion of elderly persons' homes have illumination levels markedly below the levels recommended in the Code (see Table 10.1). Levitt's subjects were felt to be a typical unselected group of elderly people, with no particular visual handicaps. A few did mention minor reading difficulties at home but had not associated it with inadequate lighting and had given no thought to lighting levels at all.

Patients in the Silver *et al.* study had impaired acuities between 6/18 and 1/60. Distance and near acuity and performance within the eye clinic was compared with that achieved within the person's own home. The homes in general proved

Table 10.1 Survey of the lighting in the homes of twenty old-age pensioners, compared to the CIBS Code recommendations. *After Levitt, J., 'Lighting for the Elderly – An Optician's View'. Proceedings of the Light for Low Vision Symposium, 1978.*

	Illuminance (lux)					
	Levitt study 1978		CIBS Standard service recommendation		CIBS recommendation for old people (50–100% increase)	
	Range	Mean	Casual reading	Prolonged reading, sewing	Casual reading	Prolonged reading, sewing
Near task living-room	30–240	100	150	300	225–300	460–600
Working surface, kitchen	35–180	90		300		450–600
Bedhead, bedroom	5–350	90		150		225–300
Centre tread, stairs	5–180	20		100		150–200

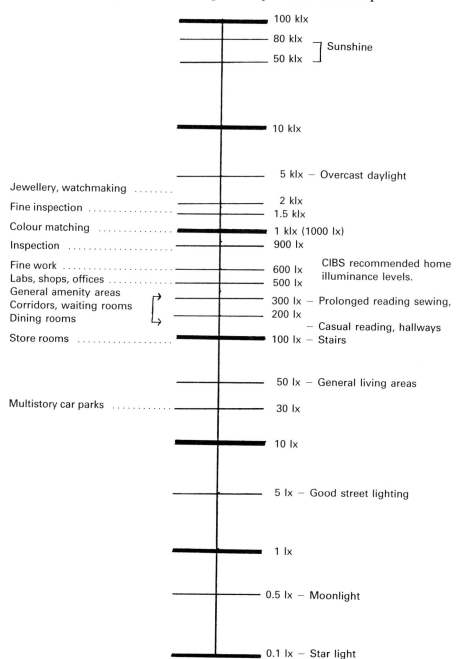

Fig. 10.2 Examples of comparative illuminance levels. Derived from the CIBS Code for Internal Lighting (1984).

to be very badly illuminated, giving rise to inferior visual performance in the great majority of patients.

Normal age related changes predominantly involve the pupil and crystalline lens. Senile miosis reduces the amount of light reaching the retina and retards the speed and ability of the eye to adapt to varying light levels. Lens sclerosis increases a person's susceptibility to glare and reduces total light transmission with a selectively greater loss of the short (blue) wavelengths.

It is very informative to listen to the comments of elderly patients who have undergone unilateral cataract extraction while retaining reasonable vision in the other eye. The sudden transformation in the colour perception of the aphakic or pseudo-phakic eye is frequently described with enormous pleasure. Remarks such as 'the house looked as if it had been repainted'; 'everything is vivid and brightly coloured with my "new" eye'; and so on, indicate very dramatically how large scale is the loss of light and colour perception induced by perfectly normal ageing effects.

Optometrists could provide a valuable service to older patients by drawing attention to the importance of good lighting at home. The lighting should take account of reduced transmission levels, slower rates of adaptation, and the greater likelihood of discomfort glare. A high proportion of visually impaired people are elderly. Specific degenerative or pathological changes are then super-imposed on the normal age-related effects.

Positioning of light sources and windows should be considered in relation to the person's work areas and normal lines of sight. Windows can be a major glare source. Objects positioned immediately next to a window are difficult to see because of the severe contrast between the light levels of the window and adjacent wall areas − a form of disability glare. Reflections of windows or light sources off shiny surfaces can also impair vision − veiling reflections (Fig. 10.3).

The common arrangement of positioning sink and draining board immediately under a window can cause difficulty for many visually impaired people. Another example of poor room organisation is to position a decorative table lamp on top or at the side of the television. It may look very attractive, but when switched on forms a glare source directly in the line of sight, reducing contrast and screen visibility.

When advising on general lighting requirements, the aim should be to remove large differences in light levels both within and between rooms. Spot lights giving a pattern of strongly highlighted and relatively shadowed areas may be striking and original to normally sighted people, but totally confusing to someone with impaired sight. A more even level of illumination is to be preferred. It need not necessarily be of very high intensity in general living areas as long as it is supplemented by good local task lighting as appropriate. Rather higher illumi-nance levels are needed in areas containing safety hazards such as stairs or in the vicinity of cookers and fires.

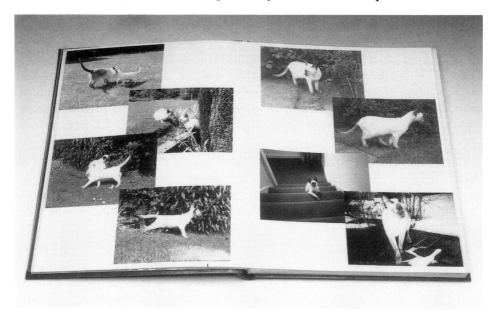

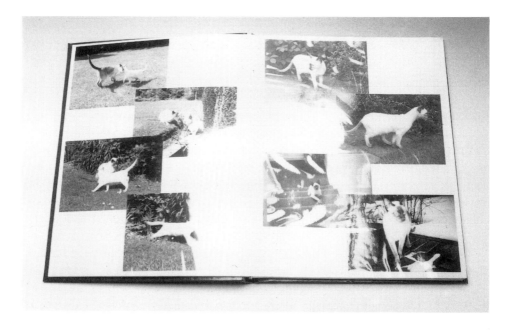

Fig. 10.3 Effect of veiling reflections on legibility illustrating the importance of correct positioning of light sources.

Fluorescent lights should be considered for kitchens. Objections to fluorescent lights at home as being 'too cold and clinical' are outdated. Fluorescent tubes are available coated with different phosphors giving a range of colour sensation from the cold 'north daylight' colour-matching tubes to deluxe warm white tubes; the latter closely resemble tungsten light by emphasising yellows and subduing blues.

10.1.3 Local lighting

Well thought-out general lighting should be supplemented by local lighting in specific activity areas such as the kitchen, or at any particular place in the house where the person habitually reads or works. Studies examining the relationship between illumination and near vision performance in visually impaired subjects emphasise the importance of high, controlled levels of light.

Sloan *et al.* (1973) and Silver (1976) suggest that people with macular disease benefit from very high levels of illumination, often well above 1000 lux. Julian (1984) used fluorescent lamps for both the general room illumination and specific task lighting in a study of the visual performance of 27 partially sighted people. He allowed people to adopt their normal reading posture. A wide variation in age and pathology of his subjects predicably produced a wide variation in individual results, but the overall pattern showed clearly that visual performance was enhanced by increased illuminance. As an average, increasing illuminance from 50 lux to 600 lux improved performance from N24 to N15.

The lighting codes recommend 450−600 lux for detailed or prolonged near vision tasks for elderly people at home. The magnitude of the problem is illustrated by the findings of an average illuminance of 100 lux (Levitt, 1978) and 177 lux (Silver *et al.*, 1978) in the reading areas in the homes of the volunteer subjects and patients surveyed.

Light from comparatively small sources conforms to the inverse square law, i.e.: halving the distance to the light source gives rise to a fourfold increase in the illuminance falling on a surface (Table 10.2). Thus in the colloquial phraseology employed with patients 'a low powered light close to your book is much better than a strong light on the ceiling'. This information is characteristically followed by the instruction to 'get an Anglepoise-type light and sit with it shining over your shoulder'.

John Collins of the Partially Sighted Society memorably describes this advice as being likely to give rise to the 'burnt-ear syndrome'! A super phrase which highlights one of the major drawbacks of tungsten-filament fittings, namely the very substantial heat output which is present even with low wattage bulbs.

As an alternative to the normal lamps there are a number of 'cool' low wattage adjustable fluorescent lamps available (Fig. 10.4). In common with all fluorescent fittings they have to have control gear and are significantly more expensive than

Table 10.2 Illuminance from tungsten filament bulbs, measured on the major axis at 40 cm and 1 m distance when mounted in Anglepoise reading lamps (after Gill & Silver (1982)).

Anglepoise mounting	Illuminance (lux)	
	40 cm dist.	1 m dist.
Clear and pearl bulbs		
60 W	460−600	70−110
100 W	900−1000	160−170
Spot-light reflector bulb		
60 W	3800	600

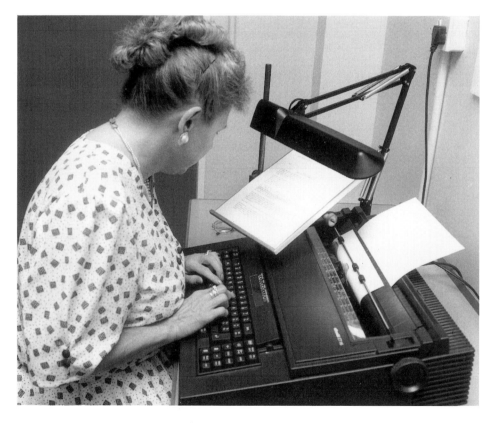

Fig. 10.4 Luxo T88 11 W, cool fluorescent lamp in use with reading stand. Correct lamp position for optimum task illumination. (Lamp available from Partially Sighted Society, Thousand & One Lamps Ltd or LVA Ltd.)

the equivalent tungsten filament unit. In use, however, fluorescent tubes are cheaper to run and have a much longer life than tungsten bulbs. Their great advantage is that they provide a much more intense, even illumination over a larger area, without heat. It is possible to sit much closer to the lamp and to handle and adjust it safely even after it has been in use for a considerable time. Adjustable lamp covers generally have reflective inner surfaces further to improve the lamps' efficiency.

Many visually handicapped people, especially if using spectacle-mounted optical aids, have to adopt an abnormally short working distance. A major difficulty is often physically to get the light onto the object without blocking and shadowing it with the patient's own hands or head. The size and heat production from a tungsten filament lamp tend to limit the options with regard to its positioning. The different size, shape and 'cool' nature of these fluorescent tubes means that it is often possible to position the lamp as shown in Fig. 10.4, i.e.: between the person's eyes and the object. The advantages of the fluorescent lamp are likely to far outweigh the drawback of the extra cost for any person doing prolonged close work.

Nevertheless, at present most people are likely to use some form of conventional tungsten bulb lamp. The effect on acuity produced by varying the distance of the lamp from the print should be clearly demonstrated to patients – several times, if necessary! A demonstration is most important since it creates a much greater impact than can possibly be achieved by a verbal description.

In fact the 'over the shoulder' position is not comfortable, since in addition to the possibility of singed ear, the lamp forms a bright, unpleasantly distracting glare source at the edge of the visual field. Positioning the lamp directly above the patient's face should also be avoided.

The lamp fitting should, if possible, be positioned further forward than the plane of the person's face so that the eyes are screened from any direct glare from the light source. Angling the lamp relative to the page also ensures that disturbing veiling reflections do not reduce contrast and interfere with vision (Fig. 10.5).

Local lighting for work surfaces

Small lights are sometimes fitted below kitchen wall-units to illuminate the work surface beneath. The positioning of such lights may need to be adjusted if they are to meet the needs of a visually impaired user (Fig. 10.6).

A normally-sighted person usually carries out manual tasks at a comfortable arm's-reach, i.e. approximately 40–50 cm range. The visually impaired person must frequently bend down to get get much closer to the object of interest. The 'kitchen-unit' situation provides an example of the way lighting design

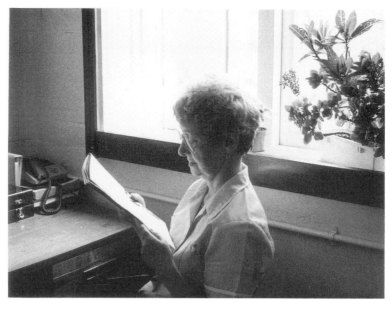

Fig. 10.5 (a) Consulting room demonstration of correct position when reading in natural light by a window. Sitting, half turned, with back to window, gives strong, unshadowed light across the page from the side, while eliminating direct glare into the eyes.

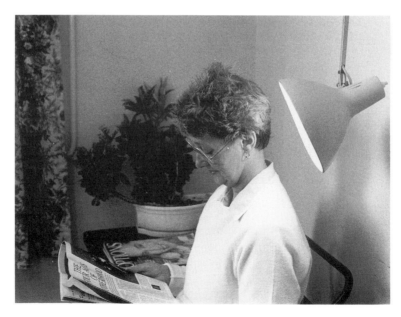

Fig. 10.5 (b) Incorrect positioning of local light: light is too far back, producing an unpleasant glare source in the peripheral visual field. Heat output from a tungsten bulb is also likely to be uncomfortable.

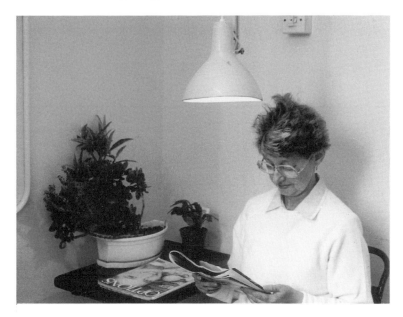

Fig. 10.5 (c) Unsatisfactory: light source directly above the face and page is still liable to form a glare source. Images of the light bulb are also likely to be reflected off shiny paper, directly into the reader's eyes.

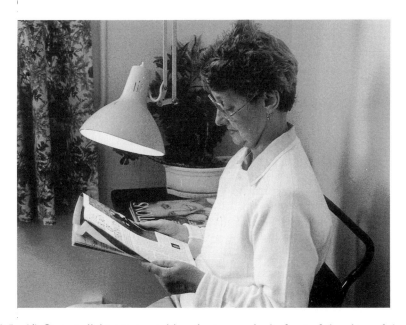

Fig. 10.5 (d) Correct: light source positioned, at an angle, in front of the plane of the face. Eyes are in relative shadow, reflections are unlikely to be a problem and the close proximity of the light source and page provides maximum illumination on to the print.

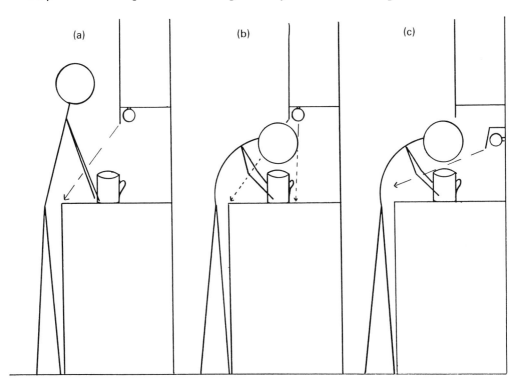

Fig. 10.6 Example of a kitchen work-area lighting design, modified for a visually impaired user. Light position which is satisfactory for a normally sighted person (a) may give unacceptable shadowing because of the different head position of a visually impaired user (b). Correctly repositioned and screened (c).

and layout may need to be individually tailored to the persons particular requirements.

Directional lighting

Visibility of some industrial tasks and some craft-type hobbies such as engraving, carving, etc., may benefit from directional local lighting.

'Modelling' is the ability of light to reveal solid form. It varies with the intensity and direction of the incident light. Practical trials may be necessary to determine to what extent modelling might assist perception of task detail. Small, single sources produce strong shadows and harsh modelling; larger sources give softer shadows and flatter modelling effects.

Surface characteristics, texture and relief are emphasised by a strong flow of light nearly parallel to the surface. In some instances the position of the light source may be more critical than its intensity. When considering directional lighting, it is advisable to reduce the possibility of discomfort glare by reducing the reflectance of surrounding surfaces, e.g. by introducing a dark, matt background behind the object.

Table 10.3 lists the properties of the general types of light sources. As with optical aids, the practitioner should be aware of the various alternatives in order to demonstrate the effects to patients – the final choice will again rest with the patient.

10.2 Colour and contrast

10.2.1 General considerations

The overall level of illumination in a room depends not only on the luminaires, but also on the colour and reflectance of the furnishings, and wall, ceiling and floor surfaces. If the aim was purely to reduce electricity costs to a minimum, one would construct an all-white room with high reflectance glossy surfaces. This would obviously be a disaster for a visually impaired person. The visual system, perception in general, is a response to differences between objects – not

Table 10.3 Summary of the characteristics of major alternative designs of light source

Lamp type	Efficacy (lumen/watt)	Colour appearance	General Description
Incandescent			
Tungsten-filament	11 (ave.)	Warm; emphasises yellows	Inert gas in a glass bulb. Small, cheap Easily dimmed, Life 1000 hours. High heat output.
Tungsten-halogen	21 (ave.)	Warm; emphasises red, subdues blues	Silica bulb containing halogen or halides, increased life and/or efficacy. Life 2000 hours. Gets hot.
Fluorescent			
Low pressure mercury vapour tubes	35–55 (ave.)	Cool: e.g. colour matching, intermediate, or warm. Colour determined by choice of phosphor coating.	Immediate light output when switched on. Light output affected by ambient temperature. Needs control gear. Min. heat output. Life 7500 hours.
High pressure discharge tubes			
Mercury based	50–70 (ave.)	Intermediate	Warm-up time approximately 5 minutes re-ignition delay approximately 10 minutes
Sodium based	95–105 (ave.)	Warm: strong yellow light subdues blue	Warm-up time approximately 2 minutes, re-ignition delay approximately 1 minute.

merely to 'light' as such. Colour can be used constructively to emphasise differences between objects while ensuring that the total area of dark colour within a room is comparatively small (Jay, 1978).

High reflectance colours (white, pale grey, cream, lemon, etc.) reflect up to 75% of the light falling on them. This reflected light then falls on other surfaces. Dark colours may reflect as little as 5% of the incident light, with the remaining 95% being absorbed.

Gloss paint, despite being easier to clean, should be avoided if possible for large surfaces such as ceilings and the upper parts of walls. The glossy surface reflects light sources with resultant irritating glare and shiny, glittery patches. Eggshell or matt paint or wallpaper is to be preferred. Light levels can be considerably enhanced if windows are kept clean and net curtains discarded whenever possible. Jay (1978) states that, if essential for privacy, the lightest possible net should be used and it must be clean! He states that the light transmission is of the order of 70% through clean net, but falls to 15−20% through dirty net.

10.2.2   Orientation

Light sources and windows are very useful orientation clues for a severely visually impaired person. Paint used on window frames and surrounds should be white or a very light colour to soften the contrast between the bright sky and the frame and room interior.

The overwhelming majority of visually impaired people retain some colour sense even though it may be severely compromised by the ocular pathology. Subtle variations in colour and shade are unlikely to be perceived. Strong, saturated colours are likely to be needed which might well look rather startling or garish to the normally-sighted. Providing these limitations are kept in mind colour can be used to give orientational and visual clues.

Walls and ceilings, as already indicated, should generally be light coloured. However, if both are a similar colour with no differentiation between them, the visually impaired person will find they tend to merge, one into the other. A contrasting colour frieze round the top of the wall and a discernably different colour floor-covering will help to define the size and shape of the room.

A cream door in a cream wall effectively disappears. Paint the door in a strong colour and it is immediately visible. If that idea can be extended to painting the doorframe in another contrasting colour it begins to be easier to judge if the door is open or closed. The door handle should be large and brightly coloured or set in a contrasting coloured panel.

Positioning a brightly coloured stripe or rail at waist height along a corridor wall will help define the physical size and shape of the area. A featureless, light-coloured wall is liable to merge into the general blur for someone with impaired sight − with painful consequences!

10.2.3 General activity areas

On a smaller, but no less important, scale, the colour of individual objects can be a valuable visual aid. This applies particularly in the kitchen. It is necessary to give patients specific examples of how to use colour contrast. For example:

- Different coloured containers for similar coloured things e.g. tea and coffee; sugar and flour, etc. Better still if the containers can be different sizes and/ or shapes as well as different colours.
- Chopping boards with a light-coloured side and a dark-coloured side. The person uses whichever is appropriate to contrast with the food being prepared.
- Dark-coloured table cloth or place mats if the china is light-coloured and vice versa.
- A range of different coloured plates, casseroles, pans, etc., to give contrast depending on the predominant colour of the food being placed on them.
- Coloured rather than clear glasswear.
- Different colours for sugar basin, milk jug, cups and saucers and so on.

The list of ideas and suggestions is endless. It is not necessary to embark on a large-scale spending spree. Normally sighted relatives and friends can often transform existing objects with the application of a coat of paint or strips of bright reflective sticky tape, once you have started them thinking along the right lines.

An elderly person may be unable or unwilling to undertake major decorative changes at home, but this type of small scale modification to routine objects can be accomplished comparatively easily and can make a big difference to the ease of performance of everyday tasks and activities.

Unlike elderly patients, parents of a visually impaired child are often very receptive to constructive suggestions on home environment lighting and design. They frequently feel very helpless when confronted by the fact that their child cannot see very well. They are anxious to make the best possible provision for the child but have no idea what to do or where to start.

Once the parents have grasped the basic ideas of light, colour, contrast, size and texture being active aids to vision they will take account of these factors when planning decoration at home and when buying both toys and general household objects.

10.2.4 Detailed near vision tasks

Performance on detailed near vision tasks increases with increasing illumination, following the law of diminishing returns, until the performance saturates, i.e. no further improvement occurs when illumination is increased (Boyce, 1978). Fig. 10.7 indicates that performance is influenced not only by the illumination

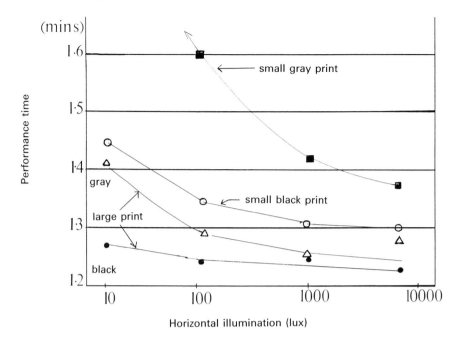

Fig. 10.7 Variation in the time taken for copy typing a printed passage by young observers at different illumination levels. Performance improves as illumination increases until performance saturates. Contrast also affects performance. High contrast print is read more quickly than the same size low contrast print. After P.R. Boyce (1978) 'The Relationship Between the Performance of Visual Tasks and the Lighting Conditions', *Light for Low Vision Symposium*.

level, but by the colour contrast of the task. Black print can be read more quickly than the same size grey print. The difference in performance is greatest in poor illumination. These results were obtained from normally sighted young observers. Extrapolating to consideration of a visually impaired person, it is clear that documents, duplicated work-sheets, etc., need to have a high contrast. One must endeavour to avoid the 'blue ink on blue paper' situation.

Teachers, work colleagues, family and friends all need 'educating' in the need for good contrast in correspondence or printed texts. A letter written in black fibre pen may be read with comparative ease; however, the same thing written in pencil would be more difficult to decipher.

10.3   Summary

Skilful use of lighting, colour and contrast can make a tremendous difference to the efficiency with which a visually impaired person can use residual vision.

It is essential to demonstrate the effect of good and bad lighting on near vision performance – not just to talk about it! Ideas for using colour contrast as a visual aid are easily understood by patients and supporters alike.

Suggestions about modifying household articles, kitchen utensils, containers and so on, are generally well received. Family and friends are pleased to find there is something practical and positive that they can do to help.

Obviously it is very important that visually impaired people get this type of advice. However, the underlying principles are relevant to all elderly people in view of the normal age-related changes within the eye as a whole, and the crystalline lens in particular.

Questions

1 What are the normal age related changes in the eye which affect light and colour perception?
(See section [10.1.2].)

2 Differentiate between disability and discomfort glare.
(See section [10.1.1].)

3 Discuss good lighting principles as applied to the homes of elderly and/or visually impaired people.
(See section [10.1.2].)

4 When talking to patients. How do you explain and demonstrate the importance and effect of local lighting on detailed tasks?
(See section [10.1.3].)

5 Where should a local light source be positioned for maximum effect when reading?
Are there any alternatives to conventional tungsten-filament bulbs?
(See section [10.1.3].)

6 What advice would you give to the parents of a visually impaired child with regard to the use of light and colour in the home?
(See section [10.2.3].)

7 Give a few practical examples of the use of colour contrast as a visual aid within the home.
(See section [10.2.3].)

8 While on the subject of colour and contrast, any suggestions for enhancing the visibility of the television picture for an elderly person with macular problems?
(Chapter 11, Case 2).

CHAPTER 11

Example Case Histories

Case 1   Congenital cataract

Diagnosis
Congenital cataract, registered partially sighted. Youngest and most severely affected member of a large family in whom congenital cataracts show a strong dominant inheritance pattern.

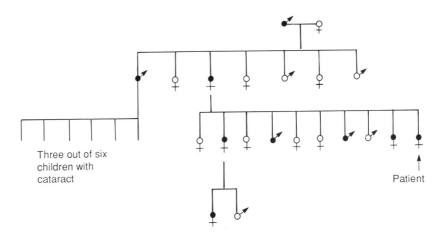

Fig. 11.1

Undilated

Cataract obscures whole pupil area; there is no visible retinoscopy reflex.
In bright light: Binoc. vision 2/60, N12.
In dim light: Visions RE 6/60, LE 6/36, N10.

Dilated

A narrow zone of clear lens is visible surrounding the cataract, R and L.
R$_x$ +2.00DS R and L, VA(R) 6/24, VA(L) 6/36.

Mother and cousins have had cataract extractions. The family view is that their vision is on the whole worse than that of the unoperated family members!

School authorities were very helpful. They had, after all, had her nine brothers and sisters as pupils, so were no strangers to the family visual problems! With some additional teaching support the child coped quite well at her local junior school before moving onto a mainstream secondary school.

The girl now works as a care assistant in an old people's home.

LVA management

Age 6 years: Tinted spectacles.

Age 9 years: Complains of occasional difficulty with print. Loaned a 5× stand magnifier (N5).

Age 10 years: Uses magnifier at home. Wants glasses for school for reading and writing as 'magnifier is too slow and the stand gets in the way'.

Ordered Franklin split bifocals R and L $\dfrac{+2.00 \text{ dist}}{+10.00 \text{ DS with 4 B in}}$

Achieves N8 binoc adequate for junior school level books.

Age 11 years: Glasses broken. Were used all day at school — 'need to be a bit stronger'.

Replaced with R and L $\dfrac{+2.00 \text{ DS distance}}{+12.00 \text{ DS with 6B in}}$ N6/N5

Age 12 years: Very self-conscious about appearance of spectacles. Franklin bifs replaced with Sola LVA bifs 38 seg decentred in as far as possible.

Age 13 years: Has tried elder brother's eye drops — found them helpful. Atropine sulphate 0.25% od (once a day) for pupil dilation. Binoc. VA 6/36 in dim and bright light.

Age 14–17 years: Continued with pupil dilation. Developed an allergic-type reaction to atropine; all other mydriatic options tried but found to be less satisfactory since the dilating effect wore off too quickly. Allergy recently discovered to be an sensitivity reaction to benzalkonium chloride. Now very happy with unpreserved atropine sulphate 0.25%. Still uses bifocal spectacles but also has a pair of full aperture +12.00D reading glasses for a larger field of view.

She always refused to use a monocular at school, but has been 'converted' by the desire for independence — and the practical problem of getting to work. Bus drivers were abusive if she stopped the wrong bus, and she kept being late for work when the correct bus sailed past the bus stop! Now uses 8 × 20 extra-short focus monocular.

Case 2   Dry, atrophic senile macular degeneration

Diagnosis

Dry, atrophic bilateral macular degeneration. Minor amounts of lenticular opacity R and L.

Age: 72

History: Widow. Lives alone. Slow, gradual deterioration of vision over two to three years. General health fair, 'bit of arthritis in hands'. Manages her household activities adequately; 'never been a big reader', but irritated by inability to read own post properly; can't see prices in shops and the TV picture is blurred.

Present R_x:
     R $-1.50/+0.75 \times 125$ 6/36   Add $+3.50$ N12/N10
     L $-2.00/+1.00 \times 85$ 6/24+

LVA assessment

(1) No improvement possible in spectacles for distance use. Reassured that watching TV is not harmful to her eyes. Told simply to sit closer to the set and experiment with the colour and contrast settings. (Many visually impaired people are more comfortable with a high contrast black and white set, rather than a normal balance colour setting.)

(2) Shown the effect of improving task lighting. Reading acuity improved from a poor N10 to a reasonable N8 with existing glasses. However, she has no local lighting at home, and being on income support, is unlikely to purchase appropriate types of adjustable lamps.

Shown low power hand and stand lenses and the effect of high-add reading glasses. Achieved N6 with a $+8.00$D add and good light, but totally rejected the idea of 'holding things right at the end of my nose'. Stand lenses were preferred to hand mags for prolonged use.

Issued with a 3× illuminated stand lens – N5 easily.

(3) Shopping/prices: loaned a small, non-aspheric 4.4 × Windsor hand lens to use for prices. Advised to hang it on a long cord round her neck when shopping. The magnifier is then always handy, even with her hands full of shopping, she doesn't actually have to carry it round in her hand, and it will not get lost so easily.

Patient will be reviewed annually.

Case 3   Proliferative diabetic retinopathy

Diagnosis: Severe proliferative diabetic retinopathy.

Age: 39 years.

Occupation: Sales assistant, DIY/hardware store.

History: Insulin dependent diabetic since age of 12 years. Referred to Eye Department Retinal Unit, aged 29 years, VA 6/6 R and L, but with proliferative retinopathy and bilateral new vessel formation. Massive retinal photocoagulation R and L, but lost the vision in his left eye four years later due to an inoperable traction detachment following repeated vitreous haemorrhages.

Present situation:
   Registered partially sighted.
   R −3.50/+1.75 × 150 6/24 Add +4.00, N14.
   L NPL (no perception of light)
   Field: generalised restriction, patchy.
   Colour vision: poor discrimination.

Assessment

(1)   General distance vision: relies on lifts to and from work. Will travel alone, but monocular, severely impaired field is a major hazard when judging traffic speeds, etc. Outdoors, glare is an increasing problem as recurrent vitreous haemorrhages render his ocular media more and more hazy. Indoors, he moves around quite freely. Uses clear spectacles indoors, with Rodenstock Lambda 660 brown block filter 10% transmission lenses, with brown tinted sideshields, outdoors.

(2)   Work: needs to see poor contrast, duplicated delivery notes, catalogues and invoices. Anxious to avoid cosmetically noticeable units when dealing with customers. Lighting poor in storerooms and office area, so has obtained two fluorescent adjustable desk lamps. These enable him to read reasonable quality print. This is supplemented by a 4× Eschenbach stand magnifier for poor quality items, and a 4× illuminated stand lens for occasions when 'he has to go to the work, rather than bringing the work to the light'.

(3)   Hobbies: carpentry, DIY (Fig. 11.2): Unconcerned about the cosmetic appearance, needs to be able to use both hands with a reasonable working distance. A 4× Eschenbach telescopic unit gives the required acuity and working distance. The monocular 'clip' unit would not remain stable enough over his spectacle lens, so the integral binocular, frame mounted unit was preferred, even though the patient has vision only in one eye.

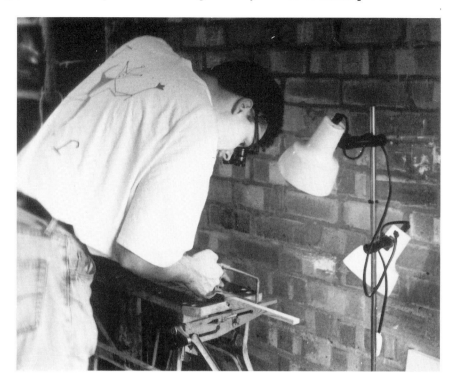

Fig. 11.2 Eschenbach binocular 4× near vision telescopic spectacles for DIY carpentry in garage workshop.

Review every six months, or more frequently if vitreous haemorrhages disrupt vision.

Case 4 Ty-neg albinism

Diagnosis: Ty-neg oculo-cutaneous albinism.

Age: 25 years.

Occupation: works in London advertising agency after obtaining an English degree.

History: First seen, aged 12 years. Pupil at a direct-grant grammar school.

> R +3.00/+4.00 × 95 6/60 Photochromic lenses.
> L +2.50/+4.00 × 95 6/60
> R/ACS 20° Nystagmus, no abnormal head posture.
> Colour vision normal; mild photophobia.

At that stage, girl was using a 5× stand mag (N5) and a fixed-focus 8 × 24 monocular for the blackboard.

Age 14 years: Fitted with tinted soft lenses with a clear pupil.
Acuity unchanged (6/60 binoc), but subjectively a significant reduction in photophobia. The soft lenses have been replaced, initially with polymethylmethacrylate material, and currently with medium grey gas permeable lenses (necessary due to peripheral vascularisation). Binocular acuity 6/36 with current lenses, with a marked improvement in contrast sensitivity when compared to spectacle correction.

LVA management

For a long time the girl refused to consider any alteration in the stand magnifier as she was comfortable and secure with what she was used to. She was eventually persuaded to try spectacle mounted units after her O-levels.

Present situation:
Distance: 8 × 20 extra short focus monocular. This adjustable monocular had replaced the fixed-focus style when she went to university to enable her to read notice boards, etc; (distance 6/6).

Intermediate: Eschenbach 3× spectacle mounted telescope.
Gives N10 at 2 to 3 metres − used for VDU and computer graphic display screen.
Near: Near VA (with CLs) − N8 at 10 cm LE, 'hard work'.
Prolonged reading − R. Afocal; L. 4× COIL Hyperocular (N5 at 8 cm)
For writing and art work − R and L +8.00DS, one pair full aperture, blended aspherics into a fashion frame, plus the same R_x into a fashion half-eye frame. Reduced R_x gives N8 equivalent at 12 to 14 cm range. Spectacles used selectively depending upon the need for simultaneous distance vision.

Reviewed 'as and when something new crops up that she can't manage to see'!

Case 5 Ty-neg albinism

Diagnosis: Ty-neg oculo-cutaneous albinism.

Age: mid-40s.

Occupation: Teacher, head of specialist unit for visually impaired children.

History:
Basic R_x R +6.00/+3.50 × 100 6/60   Near N14
L +5.50/+3.50 × 90 6/60
RDS approximately 25°. Gross nystagmus, very photophobic.

LVA Management

Distance: tinted R_x worn constantly, one pair with standard brown 20% LTF lenses and a pair with Rodenstock Lambda 660 block filter lenses. He finds the block filter lens to be more effective overall, with regard to the glare/photophobia problems, but its greater colour distortion is sometimes disturbing. He therefore selects the tint appropriate to the activity/lighting conditions concerned. 8×20 extra short focus monocular (6/5). Used 'occasionally'.

Work:

(1) While teaching, large print size and large handwriting of young pupils enable him to cope visually during actual lesson periods.

(2) Work preparation/reading – spectacle mounted Keeler LVA12 bifocal. Full distance R_x R and L (untinted), with $5\times$ LVA12 bifocal button cemented onto the left lens. Gives N5 at 7 cm.

(3) During meetings uses a black fibre pen for own note taking, and normal distance spectacles with a $6\times$ hand-held magnifier to read documents, etc. This enables him to retain a more conventional working distance, while retaining optimum distance vision and field of view for interaction with colleagues seated round him.

    Telescopic spectacle mounted units have been tried as an alternative to the high plus lens bifocal design. They were rejected on the grounds of the inferior field of view, and interestingly, because the patient was most uncomfortable with the longer working distance. Having, as he said, 'spent all my life rubbing my nose on the page, sitting back away from things feels highly abnormal'.

Reviewed 'as necessary' ... spends a lot of time in the eye department on behalf of his pupils; almost an honorary member of staff.

Case 6 Stargardt's juvenile macular dystrophy

Diagnosis: Stargardt's juvenile macular dystrophy.

Age: 20 years.

Occupation: University student.

History: First seen at age 11 years, transferred to local special school. Eye problem recognised at age 8 years; both older brothers also have macular dystrophy. Negligible refractive error, full field poor colour discrimination.

LVA management

Age 11 years: Vr 5/60, V1 6/60, Binoc 6/36, N12 at 10 cm.
No difficulty with distance vision (teaching methods do not use blackboard) or mobility. Difficulty with textbooks.
Assessment: Add +4.00 − N8; Add +6.00 − N6; Add +8.00 − N5;
Ordered Franklin split bifs, R & L Afocal/Add +8.00 with 5 B. in e.e.

Age 12 years: Vision worse. Binoc 6/60, N8 only with glasses.
Ordered: R. Afocal, L. Afocal with Keeler LVA 12 4X magnification (N5).

Age 13 years: Now only N8 with Keeler unit. Magnification increased to 6x, giving N5 again. Now using elder brother's 'cast-off' 8 × 24 monocular!

Age 15 years: V_r 4/60, V_1 4/60 (bl). RE now marginally better acuity than LE. Wants to be able to choose which eye to use. Frame ordered with both lenses trephined to take Keeler LVA12 unit. Magnification increased to 7x.

Age 16 years: Difficulty reading his own writing. 4× LVA12 button supplied to use in other side of existing spectacles.

Age 18 years: Going to university to read physics. Distance binocular vision 3/60, glasses battered, and wants larger reading area. Also needs to be able to read computer and VDU screens, and needs something with a longer working distance for soldering and metalwork.

Equipped with:

(1) 8 × 20 extra short focus monocular (6/7.5).
(2) Eschenbach binocular 4× spectacle mounted focussing near telescope.
(3) Reading glasses. R. Afocal, L.8× COIL hyperocular.
(4) Peak 10× light loupe (for emergencies).

Case 7 Bull's eye macular dystrophy

Diagnosis: Bull's eye macular dystrophy.

Age: 28 years.

Occupation: Industrial electronic assembly work (some of which is colour coded).

History: First assessed, aged 21 years, science student at polytechnic. Had only recently arrived in Britain from Iran. No previous ophthalmological or visual assessment. Difficulty with blackboard/lecture theatres and with departure/notice boards when travelling; cannot see some textbooks. Age of onset of visual problems unclear.

LVA management

Age 21 years:
    R − 2.50DS 6/36
    L − 2.50DS 6/24   Unaided near N10/N8 at 10 cm range.

Loaned

(1) 6 × 15 miniature binoculars (6/6 binoc).
(2) 6× COIL stand magnifier (N5).
(3) Fleximag (for laboratory practical work, leaving hands free).

Age 23 years: Distance acuity unchanged. Returned Fleximag (never used) and exchanged miniature binoculars for 8 × 30 short focus monocular which gave a larger, better illuminated field of view.

Age 28 years:
    R − 3.00DS 6/60
    L − 3.00DS 6/60   Unaided near N10 at 6 cm for short time.

Complained of increased difficulty at work. Muddling colours and unable to sustain necessary near vision levels for the working day. Uses monocular in unfamiliar surroundings. Reads with magnifier at home, but needs hands free so cannot use it at work.

Assessment: manages N5 LE, at 5 cm with a +9.00D add, but this is an unacceptably short working distance. Must have room to manipulate small electronic components. Supplied with Rayner Telecap unit; basic magnification 1.75× with a distance cap for television and a near cap +6.00D which gives a combined magnification of 5.25×. With this unit the patient could see N5 at 10 cm range. Unit fitted to the LE of frame, RE glazed with −3.00DS lens to give distance vision when patient looks up from his work.
    Colour vision was assessed with the 100 Hue test. He had an error score of RE 1019, LE 909, with a loss of discrimination across the whole spectrum.

Case 8 Disciform senile macular degeneration

Diagnosis: Disciform senile macular degeneration.

Age: 67 years.

History: Very fit retired lady who has always done a large amount of reading. Established disciform lesion LE, and has now developed a rapid onset, disciform lesion in her RE with a neovascular membrane centred on the macula, not amenable to laser treatment. Lady is very distressed by the loss of her near vision, which has been reduced from normal to N24 in the space of 6 months.

R$_x$ R. +2.00/+1.50 × 70 5/60 Add +3.00 − N24.
L. +1.50/ +2.00 × 60 2/60 Add +3.00 − N36.

LVA management

First visit: Near vision assessment with conventional direct viewing was unrewarding. An 8x magnifier still only giving approximately N12, the patient became distressed and tearful at her inability to achieve any useful vision.

Amsler chart assessment showed an area of much clearer vision to the right of fixation. Wearing her ordinary reading glasses, the patient was directed to look to the left of the words. A typoscope provided extra help in keeping her steady on the line, and with repeated reminders to keep her eyes still and move the book (i.e. steady eye strategy) near VA improved from N24 to N14.

The lady's husband was then involved to help and encourage, and with a trial frame replacing her own glasses, plus lenses added until acuity reached N10. The lady could then read a standard large print book. Book, typoscope and temporary glasses were then loaned for a three week trial/practice period.

Second visit: Lady and husband both said it was very hard work. She had frequently got upset but had persevered and could now read N10 print 'without too many mistakes'. Retesting showed that she could see some parts of N8 text, although this was still very difficult.

Permanent spectacles were ordered:
RE 4× COIL hyperocular, LE Occluded.
Lens choice to give the largest field of view, other eye occluded to eliminate confusion from the left eye.
On collection, viewing angle, working distance and the importance of correct lighting were again demonstrated and emphasised.

Such patients are seen for regular follow-up appointments. This particular lady finally managed to read N8-size library books with sufficient fluency to render it enjoyable again. She was also supplied with a 6× hand lens for reading prices when shopping. She concentrated on imagining she was looking at the left rim of the magnifier, closed her left eye, and positioned the price ticket under the centre of the lens.

Eccentric viewing was by then such a habit that she automatically looked to the left of any object of interest, whatever its distance; when crossing roads, watching TV or reading.

Case 9   Homonymous hemianopia

Diagnosis: L homonymous hemianopia with partial loss of use of left arm and leg following a stroke nine months ago.

Age: 74 years.

History: Spends a lot of time reading since walking is difficult; c/o continually missing the first section of the line and having to 'backtrack'. Also holding a book and turning the page at the same time is tricky in view of the limited use of his left hand.

> R_x R. +3.00/+0.75 × 155 6/9pt.
> L. +2.75DS 6/9+.
> Separate reading glasses, Add +3.00D − N6 binocular.

LVA management

(1) Supplementary local lighting improved acuity to N5.
(2) Typoscope with a large vertical slit (see fig. 7.2) or just a strip of black card held at the left-hand side of the print provided a reference point for the start of each line.
(3) With very limited use in his left hand he was unable to hold the book and typoscope steady. A reading stand, with fluorescent strip light positioned across the top solved the problem completely.

When last seen, he reported reading comfortably for long periods. Sometimes he still used the typoscope/card, but since he no longer had to hold the book, he usually put his finger at the left end of the line as a refixation point. This he had found preferable, particularly where the page curved along the spine of the book.

Review: GOS refraction only to keep reading R_x upto date.

Case 10   Micropthalmos, coloboma, nystagmus

Diagnosis: Micropthalmos with coloboma affecting inferior retina and choroid, encroaching onto macular area. Symmetrical right and left.

Age: 6 years.

History: First encountered as a small baby. At age three months, corneal diameter 5 mm RE, 7 mm LE; gross nystagmus; corneal reflections symmetrical. Reacted to strong light and turned head in response to 40 W bulb being moved around and switched on suddenly in an otherwise dimly lit room. No response to pen torch-size light. Cycloplegic refraction−negligible refractive error.

Age 2 years: Motor development good, walking fairly well although mother worried by his obvious difficulty in judging the position of objects around him: 'he just keeps walking until he bounces off chair/wall/door, etc.,...covered in bruises'. Acuity: approximately 2/60 (rolling balls). Home teacher and specialist education staff involved with the child.

Age 4 years: Visual ability clearly improved although only in the order of 2/60 − 3/60 on formal testing. Attends special nursery school, happy mixing with other children. Navigates well! Ran at high speed through a crowded out-patient department without falling over anyone's feet!

Age 6 years: Full formal assessment at request of school who are very anxious for guidance on print size, etc., to be used in teaching programme. Attends normal primary school with peripatetic specialist teaching support. He is starting to 'take advantage' of his vision problem and will happily tackle quite small, detailed tasks if he likes the subject matter, but says 'I can't see it' if asked to work at an uncongenial topic!

    Assessment conducted in a hospital clinic with the special education teacher present but mother (by prior arrangement) remaining outside.

Vision:
Distance: Binoc 6/60 SG (Sheridan Gardiner) with only slight abnormal head posture (turns face slightly to the left and elevates chin.)
Near: N8 size detail at end of nose, RE preferred.
General impression: single letter near vision resolving power more than adequate for print size appropriate to his age. However, he has definite scanning problems, presumably resulting from the gross nystagmus and the coloboma − induced wedge-shaped field defect encroaching on the macula. Magnification was not really indicated, but we got a very positive response to a bar magnifier with a red line through the centre. The child was still able to adopt his 'nose on page' working distance, but with the teacher positioning the red line under the print, there was a noticeable improvement in reading speed with the line aiding scanning and orientation across the page.
Colour vision was examined binocularly with the City University test. Rather to my surprise the boy identified every colour match correctly. A result, however, which did not unduly surprise the teacher, who had found the child responded quite accurately to colours in the classroom.
Peripheral field: difficult to asses accurately in view of wriggly, chatty nature of subject, but appeared full to 6 mm 'hatpin' type target. No obvious mobility problems. Rushes everywhere!

    After assessment, child set about demolishing children's play area while results discussed in full with mother. Specialist teacher will explain scanning problems to the normal class teacher, but otherwise we were very encouraged by how well child performed. 'Can't see it' will no longer be acceptable as a way of avoiding work!

Cycloplegic refraction on separate occasion—again no significant error.

Review annually, or at the request of the school.

Case 11   Ty-neg albinism in family group

Diagnosis: Ty-neg albinism.

An illustration of the typical refractive error and acuity findings associated with this eye condition follows.

An immigrant Pakistani family group in which two ty-neg albino brothers married their cousins, two ty-neg albino sisters. Currently the two couples have six children, aged between four years ten years, with refractive error and VAs as follows:

Age 10 years:
>   R +2.00/+4.00 × 90 6/36
>   L +1.00/+5.00 × 90 6/60   Bin 6/24, N6.

Occasional difficulty with some of the more 'adult' school books. Has a 4× stand lens which is kept at school and used as necessary.

Age 9 years:
>   R Plano/+5.00 × 100 6/60
>   L +0.25/+4.50 × 90 6/36   Bin 6/24−1, N6.

Age 9 years:
>   R +3.50/+6.00 × 90 6/60
>   L +4.50/+5.00 × 90 6/60   Bin 6/36, N6.

Age 7:
>   R +2.25/+3.50 × 90 6/36 (linear SG).
>   L +3.50/+3.00 × 85 6/36 Bin 6/24 pt, N8/N6.

Age 6 years:
>   R +2.25/+4.25 × 85 3/12 (Ffooks) Alt. Div. Squint.
>   L +2.00/+4.00 × 90 3/12 Bin 3/12, N10/N8.

Age 4 years:
>   R +1.50/+5.00 × 90 Binoc 3/18 SG (single letters).
>   L +1.50/+4.00 × 95 Near binoc N12.

All six children are integrated into their local primary school. Additional specialist peripatetic teaching support is available as required, but otherwise all the children cope with standard textbooks and teaching methods without undue difficulty. None of the children are photophobic. None will voluntarily wear spectacles. This has resulted predictably in cheerful, low-grade guerrilla warfare between the children on one side, and ourselves plus teachers on the other side. A ceasefire position now prevails. Glasses are retained in school and used for all classroom activities. We have abandoned any attempt to have them worn outdoors!

The oldest child shortly will move to a mainstream secondary school. She will then be issued with a distance monocular for blackboard use.

Reviewed annually.

Case 12 Severe complicated congenital ocular malformation

Diagnosis: Congenital iris/anterior segment abnormality with R. posterior pole toxocara scar. Secondary glaucoma and lenticular opacity. Registered blind.

Age: 50 years.

Occupation: Local Authority clerical officer.

Present situation:
    RE NPL.
    LE +12.50/+2.50 × 20 1/60. Aphakic, surgical complete aniridia, decompensated cornea with band keratopathy.

LVA management

Very independent lady. Travels to work, etc., by bus with the help of a guide dog. Kay.

Work: Uses a CCTV. The normal platform had to be removed from below the camera unit to allow large thick ledgers to fit underneath. Screen invariably is used in reversed polarity (i.e. white on black) mode. She can see to write under a ×10 COIL stand lens, but prefers to make her own notes, etc., by means of a 'Braille and Speak' unit. This is really a braille tape recorder. The information typed in, in braille, is converted and played back as required by means of a voice synthesiser (Fig. 9.4).

Home: Reads a limited amount with a Peak 15× light loupe, held in contact with her distance spectacles (N8 for a short time).

Hobbies: Tapestry. Keeler LVA12 bifocal unit, 9× magnification cemented onto a +15.00D carrier lens. Realistically, however, she has to restrict herself to using thick, brightly coloured wools on a very open weave fabric backing.

General mobility: The decompensated cornea gives rise to severe disability glare and disorientation problems if subjected to sudden changes in light intensity.

This arises both outdoors and within the large openplan office and multistorey office building where she works — walking into a patch of sunlight shining through a window or into light shining from an open doorway and then into a relatively dimly lit corridor, for example. Trials with various tinted clip-over lenses evinced a strong preference for the 20% LTF Lambda tint — 'much more comfortable'.

APPENDIX 1

Registration Criteria in Britain

Decisions regarding registration as a blind or partially sighted person are made by a consultant ophthalmologist who completes form BD8 in England and Wales and BPI in Scotland. The fee for completing the registration document is paid by the relevant health authority.

A.1.1 Definition of blindness

The statutory definition for the purposes of registration as a blind person under the National Assistance Act 1948, is that the person is 'so blind as to be unable to perform any work for which eyesight is essential'.

The test is not whether the person is unable to pursue his ordinary occupation or any particular occupation, but whether he or she is too blind to perform *any work* for which eyesight is essential. Only the visual conditions are to be taken into account. Other physical or mental conditions are disregarded.

The main condition to consider is the visual acuity, i.e. the best direct vision obtainable with each eye separately, or binocularly, if both eyes are present, tested by Snellen type, with appropriate spectacle correction. Regard must also be paid to other conditions set out below.

Group 1 – below 3/60 Snellen

Most people who have an acuity below 3/60 should be certified as blind. 1/18 should not be certified as blind unless there is a considerable field restriction.

Group 2 – 3/60 but below 6/60 Snellen

Certify as blind if the field of vision is very contracted. Persons should not be regarded as blind if the defect is of long standing or unaccompanied by any material contraction of the visual field, e.g. congenital nystagmus, albinism, myopia, etc.

Group 3 — 6/60 Snellen or above

A person with a visual acuity of 6/60 or better should not ordinarily be regarded as blind. Individuals may be certified as blind, however, if the field of vision is markedly contracted in the greater part of its extent, particularly if the contraction is in the lower part of the field. A person suffering from homonymous or bi-temporal hemianopia retaining central acuity of 6/18 or better is not to be regarded as blind.

Other points to be considered:

(1) Duration of visual problem: a person whose eyesight has failed recently may find it more difficult to adapt than a person with the same visual acuity whose eyesight failed a long time ago.
(2) Age of patient: an old person with a recent failure of sight cannot adapt as readily as a younger person with the same defect.
(3) It is recognised that cases may arise which are not precisely within these guidelines. In such instances the ophthalmologist may use his or her own judgement with regard to registration.

A.1.2 Definition of partial sight

There is no legal definition of partial sight. The guidelines are that a person who is not blind within the meaning of the 1948 Act may be certified partially sighted if they are 'substantially and permanently handicapped by defective vision caused by congenital defect or injury or illness'.

People certified as partially sighted are entitled to the same help from their local social services as people who are registered blind. They are not eligible for income tax concessions or Social Security benefits which are applicable only to the blind.

A person may be certified partially sighted with visual acuity levels:

(1) 3/60 to 6/60 with full field;
(2) up to 6/24 with moderate contraction of the field, opacities in the media, or aphakia;
(3) 6/18 or better if there is a gross field defect, for example, hemianopia or marked contraction of the visual field, e.g. retinitis pigmentosa or glaucoma.

A.1.3 Notes regarding children

(1) Infants and young children who have congenital ocular abnormalities leading to visual defects should be certified as partially sighted, unless they are obviously blind.

(2) Children aged four and over should be certified as blind or partially sighted according to the binocular corrected vision;

Children should be re-examined every 12 months – or more frequently if there is reason to suspect any worsening of the condition. In making recommendations about persons up to the age of 16, it should be born in mind that there are other factors which may influence local education authorities in their decision about the special education provision required.

APPENDIX 2

Statutory Provision of Assistance and Services Following Registration as a Blind or Partially Sighted Person

A.2.1 Central government services

A.2.1.1 Finance: mandatory benefits

Central government determines the financial benefits consequent upon registration. Within the UK there is no statutory blind pension. The situation is complex and liable to change with each budget or Social Security regulation amendment. Unfortunately local Inland Revenue and DSS office staff are not always consistent or up to date in their advice.

Much valuable, regularly updated advice, is available from the Royal National Institute for the Blind (RNIB) Benefits Rights office or in the BBC *In Touch* Handbook. The DSS produce a series of leaflets including FB19, 'Social Security Benefits: A Guide for Blind and Partially Sighted People', which can be obtained from local DSS offices or Citizens' Advice Bureaux.

Automatic financial benefits are only for registered blind people (*not* those registered as partially sighted) and consist of:

- A reduction of £1.25p in the cost of a TV licence. The person should take their local authority supplied 'Certificate of Blindness' with them to the post office when renewing their licence.
- A free licence for a guide dog.
- Parking and travel concessions. Registered blind people may apply to their local Social Services department for an orange windscreen badge which entitles the holder and his or her driver to park at meters free of charge. They may also park in streets with waiting restrictions and in certain instances for up to two hours on double yellow lines. Orange badges are valid throughout the country (except central London, which has its own scheme) and in a number of European countries. Concessionary fares on trains, buses and coaches are also available to the registered blind. Details available from the appropriate organisation.
- Postal concessions. There are no postal charges on braille or Moon material or on cassettes for the blind providing they carry an 'Articles for the Blind'

label (available free from the RNIB). Normal handwritten or typed letters do not qualify for postal concessions.

- Free GOS eye examinations. This is the only financial benefit with applies both to blind and partially sighted people.

Discretionary allowances for both categories include possible help with 'travel to work' costs and payment for the services of a reader at their place of work.

A.2.1.2 Income Tax

A blind person paying income tax, or whose spouse pays tax, is entitled to an increased personal allowance. This addition is currently (i.e. 1990) set at £1080 for each registered blind taxpayer in the family.

A.2.1.3 Income support/family credit

This is the system which replaced supplementary benefit in April 1988 as the State 'safety net'. Individual needs are determined by criteria based on age, family, status, disability and accommodation. This is costed out through a variety of personal allowances and special payments known as premiums.

Within the working age groups sick pay, sickness and invalidity benefits depend upon the claimant's national insurance record but blind and partially sighted people may qualify for a severe disablement allowance even if their contribution record would not normally entitle them to invalidity benefit.

All registered blind and some partially sighted people qualify for a disability premium which is beneficial when income support levels are being assessed. In addition some blind people qualify for mobility, attendance and invalid care allowances and may then be eligible for the severe disability or the child disability premiums.

Once the individual entitlement/need level has been calculated it is compared with the person's actual income. Any shortfall is the amount of income support or family credit paid.

Normally anyone over 18 years of age may apply for income support, but registered blind 16 and 17 years olds may also apply. The value of a house owned by the claimant, the first £3000 savings, the first £15 per week earned by a registered blind person and any attendance or mobility allowances are all ignored for purposes of the calculations.

A.2.1.4 Housing Benefit

People receiving income support automatically have housing costs such as rent and mortgage costs paid in full and receive a council tax rebate. People just above income support level may be eligible for housing benefit and thus help towards cost of rent and council tax (but not mortgage payments). The savings limit for housing benefit is currently (1998) set at £8000.

Blind registration is beneficial in two ways. Firstly, the disability premiums increase the 'allowable needs' level on which calculations are based. Secondly, income from other non-dependent adults, e.g. son or daughter, living in the same house, is ignored if the claimant or spouse is registered blind.

To summarise, automatic financial benefits of registration are limited and predominantly restricted to the blind. The major elements are:

(1)   Increased level of personal allowances for those paying income tax and
(2)   A more favourable level income support/family credit and housing benefit for those on a low income.

Registered partially sighted claimants may sometimes qualify for the improved social security payments.

As may be seen from this brief summary, the system of claims and allowances is complicated in the extreme. The claim forms are not available in large print, and to make matters worse, are often printed on coloured paper which further reduces legibility. It is hardly surprising that many visually impaired people fail to get the allowances to which they are entitled.

A.2.1.5 Employment

Central government in the guise of the Department of Employment (DoE) is responsible for retraining and resettlement services for visually handicapped persons seeking employment.

The DoE Training Agency (formerly the Manpower Services Commission) has responsibility for training all unemployed people. Extra provision through the Employment Rehabilitation Service (ERS) is available for assessment and specific job training for disabled people.

The Employment division of the DoE is concerned with finding jobs. Within the service are Disablement Advisory Service teams (DAS) each with one member with special responsibility for visually impaired clients. This is the Blind Persons Resettlement Officer (BPRO) or Disablement Advisor.

In England and Wales RNIB Employment Service Staff work with DAS teams predominantly in the professional and commercial field. They provide assistance in the area of initial job placement and provide an advisory service to employers and employees should visual problems arise in existing employment. Within the industrial sphere, there are Technical Consultants or Blind Persons' Training Officers who are able to provide specialized on-the-job training and technical advice on such matters as modification of machines.

Much of the Training Agency and DAS work is done in association with voluntary agencies. St Dunstans (for armed forces and auxiliary services personnel) and the RNIB centres at Torquay and Fife provide residential courses for social and vocational assessment and training. These courses concentrate on general mobility and communication skills as well as occupational requirements. Some people would then move on to specific vocational courses such as physiotherapy or computer programming, etc.

Unemployed people seeking work should automatically be referred to the local DAS team when the local authority receives the completed BD8 full or partial registration form. The individual can also make contact directly through their local Job Centre.

In addition the registered blind or partially sighted person may request the Job Centre to include their name on the Disabled Persons Register. Disabled registration is not an automatic adjunct of blind registration but can be done at the individual's request once the Job Centre has verified the visual handicap with the local authority.

Disabled registration may have some advantage in finding work since employers with an average workforce of over 20 people have a duty to employ a 3% quota of disabled people.

In other instances disabled registration may be felt to be inappropriate.

Visually handicapped school leavers considered potentially capable of obtaining open employment may join a normal Employment Training Scheme working alongside normally sighted trainees. In most instances the starting point for information is the Job Centre.

A.2.2 Local authority provision

Local authorities have a duty under section 29 of the National Assistance Act 1948, amended by the 1972 Local Government Act 'to make provision for the welfare of people substantially and permanently handicapped by illness, injury or congenital deformity'. This has always included the blind, but was specifically extended to include the partially sighted in 1974.

The legislation is interpreted to mean that blind or partially sighted persons should be given 'in their own homes or elsewhere' instruction, advice and support to enable them to overcome or minimize the effect of their disability. The local authority must either employ suitably trained staff or finance the handicapped person's attendance at a rehabilitation centre.

The provision can be broadly subdivided into the following categories.

A.2.2.1 Daily living skills

Visually impaired persons must be helped to learn to look after themselves and carry out normal daily activities. This might for example involve instruction in basic cooking, ironing, domestic chores, etc., and information regarding the many gadgets and tactile aids available.

A.2.2.2 Communication skills and mobility training

A person unable to see to read and write has a right to be offered training in alternative methods of communication and information such as touch typing, braille and Moon.

Mobility training (i.e. instructing a blind person how to move around more safely and efficiently) is now seen as an essential part of a good rehabilitation service. Unfortunately trained personnel are in very short supply. The training may relate only to moving around indoors, or progress to full long-cane techniques which require regular daily training extending over several months, but which then enable the blind person to walk arounds outdoors confidently, even in unfamiliar surroundings. A white cane banded in red reflective tape indicates that the user has a hearing defect in addition to the visual handicap.

A.2.2.3 Recreational, occupational and social activities

Historically this has been rather limited, embracing the traditional 'craft' instruction, social clubs and possibly support for homeworker schemes.

However, more recently the Chronically Sick and Disabled Persons Act 1970 has broadened the duties and responsibilities laid on local authorities. When considered necessary, the authority must provide:

(1) Within a person's home, practical help and physical modifications and adaptations (e.g. better lighting) to minimise the effects of the disability. This may include the provision of a telephone and radio, television or other recreational facilities.
(2) Within the community, educational and recreational facilities, e.g. libraries, lectures, sports facilities. It must ensure the disabled person has adequate access to such facilities, including the provision of transport as necessary.
(3) Assistance with the provision of outings and holidays.

APPENDIX 3
Non-statutory Organisations, Services and Facilities for the Visually Impaired

Patients who are registered blind or partially sighted hopefully should be supplied with information by the local authority social services staff working with the visually impaired. The statutory system is very stretched and many people do regretably slip through the net. In addition there are large numbers of people who do not qualify for registration but who nevertheless are experiencing significant visual problems in their daily lifes. Relatives and friends also often appreciate information and advice to enable them effectively to support the person with the vision problem.

For all these reasons it is very helpful if optometrists have some knowledge of the range of non-statutory voluntary agencies and services which exist both nationally and in their local area. Addresses can then be provided and patients and families made aware of facilities which might be of interest or assistance to them.

A.3.1 Voluntary organisations, information and support groups

A.3.1.1 Royal National Institute for the Blind (RNIB)

The RNIB is the largest of the voluntary organisations concerned with blind and visually impaired people. It has a wide ranging involvement in all aspects of education, employment, and welfare services as they affect the visually impaired person.

A network of RNIB specialist advisors and centres located throughout the country provides a local service to individuals, schools and employers. Many more services are administered centrally from the RNIB London headquarters.

The organisation also produces an illustrated catalogue, *'RNIB Games and Equipment,* which contains a large number of examples of everyday household articles, such as clocks, cooking aids, card and board games, etc. which have been modified for blind or visually impaired users. Items in the catalogue may be purchased directly from the RNIB.

The Institute is a valuable source of information for professional and patient alike. It produces an extensive range of leaflets and information packs which are generally available in a choice of standard or large print, braille or cassette versions. Information and advice on general, non-medical, queries is frequently available directly to telephone callers.

A.3.1.2 Partially Sighted Society

Founded in 1973, it is concerned with the welfare of people of all ages with poor sight. It has local self-help groups throughout the country and produces a bi-monthly magazine, *Oculus*. The society will give advice and information to members or non-members on any aspect of partial sight, and has a catalogue of lamps and aids suitable for those with some residual vision.

The society runs low vision training courses for interested professionals and is particularly keen to promote a multidisciplinary approach to the provision of low vision services to improve the quality of life for visually impaired people.

A.3.1.3 *In Touch*: radio programme and handbook

A BBC Radio 4 weekly programme of news, comment and information for visually impaired people. Associated with the programme in an off-air phone-in, enabling listeners to acquire additional information and also to pass on comments or ideas which might be of interest or help to other listeners. The *In Touch* team produce a quarterly bulletin summarising broadcast information. Sadly, the regularly updated handbook has been discontinued. Both the bulletin and handbook are available in print, braille, Moon and audio-cassette versions.

The programme and associated publications contain a wealth of information on all aspects of everyday living for the visually handicapped person. The handbook is an invaluable reference book for professionals and visually handicapped persons and their families. Old editions are still very useful if you can acquire one.

A.3.1.4 Disabled Living Foundation (DLF)

The DLF is a charity, partly funded by the DSS, concerned with all disabilities, mental, physical and sensory. The Foundation aims to reduce the handicap imposed by any disability by providing information on non-medical solutions to the daily living problems resulting from the disability.

Information is available to anyone, by post, telephone or by personal visit to the Foundation's Aids Centre in London. Resource Centres, not run by the DLF, but based on similar lines are available in most major cities. These centres provide opportunities to try out aids for all types of disability in circumstances which approximate to those obtaining at home or in the workplace.

The DLF itself has a specialised visual handicap advisory service which produces information and teaching packs for professionals who deal with visually impaired people. The London centre also has a special kitchen area designed to suit the needs of people with severely impaired vision, in addition to its more general magnifier and low vision aid display.

A.3.1.5 Local associations

Many areas have their own local association or a branch of one of the larger umbrella organisations. They may provide some statutory services on behalf of the local authority or may be concerned primarily with recreational and social activities. Addresses can be obtained from local social services departments, Citizen's Advice Bureaux or from the RNIB.

The many local voluntary associations are grouped together into larger regional organisations, the South and North Regional Associations, the Wales Council and the Scottish National Federation for the Welfare of the Blind.

A.3.1.6 The National Federation of the Blind

This self-help organisation is open to all blind and partially sighted people over the age of 16. It has in the order of 30 local branches and a postal branch, and aims to offer blind people a means of voicing their views on issues which affect them – handicap allowances, schooling, employment opportunities, environmental questions and the like.

A.3.1.7 St Dunstan's

Founded in 1915, its activities are still restricted to helping individuals whose visual problems are related to their service in the Armed Forces or certain auxiliary services.

A.3.1.8 Special interest groups

There are a large number of organisations whose members share another common factor in addition to the visual impairment. The link may be religious, ethnic, occupational or related to a specific medical condition. All such associations provide members with support, fellowship and advice on specific problems, but would readily provide information to anyone contacting them.

Groups range from the very small to the national high-profile organisations such as the British Retinitis Pigmentosa Society whose active fund raising supports valuable research into the disease.

Some examples of special interest groups are given here. Addresses are given in Appendix 6.

International Glaucoma Association
The Albino Fellowship
British Diabetic Association
SENSE (Association for Deaf/Blind and Rubella Handicapped)
Association of Blind and Partially Sighted Teachers and Students
Association of Blind Chartered Physiotherapists
British Computer Association of the Blind
The Torch Trust for the Blind
British Blind Sport
Jewish Blind Society
Circle of Guide Dog Owners
Gardeners' Trust for the Blind
Macular Disease Society

These many and varied organisations and self-help groups are clearly 'consumer orientated' to the needs of the visually impaired themselves.

Professionals whose work encompasses aiding those with defective sight may be interested in joining the Association for the Education and Welfare of the Visually Handicapped. This umbrella organisation produces the thrice yearly *British Journal of Visual Impairment*, containing articles covering research and all aspects of health, welfare, education and employment related to visual disability.

A.3.2 Non-optical services and facilities for the visually impaired

A.3.2.1 Large print

(1)   Books

The Ulverscroft Press in 1964 was the first publisher commercially to produce large print books. It is still a leader in this field although there are now a number of other publishers active in this area. Isis, Landmark, Masterworks (for adult titles), and Windrush and Cornerstone (children's titles) are all divisions of Clio Press Ltd, Oxford-based producers of large print books. Chivers Press Publishers have an extensive range of titles and also act as agents for the G.K. Hall range of American large print publications. Magna Print Books include some Mills & Boon titles in their range. The National Library for the Blind 'Austin Books' series concentrates on classics and standard English works.

For obvious economic reasons the great majority of titles are fiction or 'popular' non-fiction, travel, biography, etc., with only a limited range of reference books, dictionaries, bibles, prayer and hymn books, and so on.

Books can be purchased directly from publishers but obviously the great majority are distributed via the normal library service. The Library Association takes an active interest in the provision of large print books. Essex County Library Service has compiled a catalogue (happily in large print!) of large print titles available for loan. Anyone interested in such books should enlist the help of the local librarian. The DLF has a card index of non-fiction, reference and predominantly classic titles and will deal with specific queries regarding availability of books on a particular topic.

Large print books have obvious drawbacks of size and weight which may pose problems for some users, both in terms of transporting them to and from the library and in holding them steady while reading. A reading stand may be necessary in some cases.

There is no standard format for such books. The various publishers have adopted different print sizes and styles. The larger the print, the bulkier will be the final text. For this reason some large print versions of the Bible, for example, have been split up into several volumes.

The Library Association have carried out some research into type design for the visually handicapped (Shaw, 1969). Some general indicators regarding type size, boldness and spacing did emerge but it is clearly impossible to produce a design which will be ideal for all varying types of visual problem. Individuals may therefore find they favour one publisher's layout and design rather than another.

Further information and complete catalogues are available from all the individual publishers on request.

(2)   Banks

Most major banks and some building societies produce both braille and large print versions of their information booklets and individual customer account statements. Cheque book templates are also available on request from all the various banks.

(3)   Maps

A large print map of the London Underground System is produced by the LRT Unit for Disabled Passengers. Some local associations have put together large print maps, information sheets and street guides covering their own areas.

(4)   Individual specialist requirements

Many photocopier machines have the facility to enlarge material. The PSS, the National Library for the Blind and many local associations offer an enlarging service for a person's own material. The service is normally subject to a small charge, but it is possible in this way to satisfy individual requirements for such things as sheet music, instruction manuals, rule books, scripts for actors and so on.

(5)   *Other large symbol items*

The PSS catalogue and the *RNIB Equipment and Games* Catalogue contain many examples of commercially produced items, of value to people with poor sight. Some examples are illustrated in Fig. A.3.1 and include large symbol telephones, telephone dials, clocks, playing cards, jumbo typeface typewriters, heavy lined stationery, etc.

A.3.2.2 Audio cassettes

(1)   *Talking Newspapers*

The Talking Newspaper Association of the UK co-ordinates activity in this field and produces an annual *Guide to Tape Services for the Handicapped*. This lists national and local talking newspapers, journals and reading services for the blind.

There are several hundred local groups organising local recordings of local

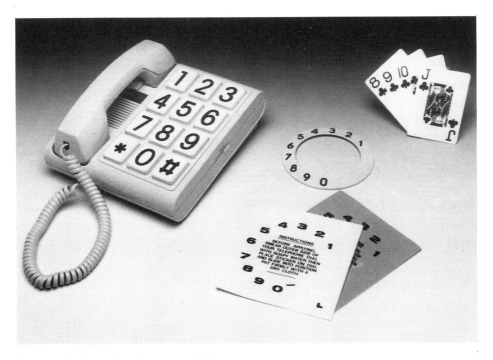

Fig. A.3.1 Examples of large symbol items.

papers on a weekly or fortnightly basis. Reading is done by volunteers onto standard cassettes.

The National organisation produces, again on standard cassettes, recordings of extracts from approximately 100 different publications. These cover national Sunday and daily papers, and many magazines including *Radio Times* and *TV Times*.

A number of specialist journals and a certain amount of religious material is available in tape form. There are also individuals and organisations who will undertake individual recordings of specific 'one-off' items. Full details of all services are available from the Talking Newspaper Association.

(2)   *Talking books*

RNIB

The RNIB has both its Talking Book Service (containing some 8000 titles) and the Student Cassette Tape Library (containing some 10 000 educational books). Membership is available to registered blind persons and anyone with defective reading vision (generally below Nl2). It is merely necessary to have the membership form endorsed to this effect by a GP, ophthalmologist, optometrist or local authority technical or mobility officer. Unfortunately, legal copyright restrictions prevent the RNIB tapes being played on standard cassette players.

The necessary specialised talking book machines are available on loan to members. The loan fee is paid either by the recipient or by the local authority. The Student Tape library is a mixture of standard and restricted cassettes. It is also possible to obtain access, via the RNIB, to the American talking book scheme. Again specialised cassette players are needed.

Calibre

This is a lending library of book recordings on tapes suitable for any standard cassette player. A catalogue of titles and membership details is available directly from the organisation.

Local library services

Local libraries are slowly expanding the range of cassettes available for loan, although unlike books, there is a small fee for cassettes.

Purchase

The numbers of commercially produced tapes available for purchase is increasing all the time. Chivers Press Publishers for example, in addition to their large print range, produce audio books for both adults and children which are available directly from the publishers or through normal retail outlets.

Combined large print books and audio tapes

Cornerstone (a division of Isis/Clio Press) have a small range of children's works comprising a combined set of a large print book and an audio cassette of the same story. The aim is for the visually impaired child to follow the printed words while listening to the story.

Individual optometrists and low vision aid clinics cannot be expected to become miniature resource centres. As with some other aspects of LVA work the aim should be to provide the basic information, ideas and addresses as appropriate. Thus, by pointing individual patients in the right direction, one hopefully will enable them to extract the items and make the contacts likely to be of value to them in their own particular circumstances.

Questions

1   What national voluntary organisations provide advice and assistance for visually impaired people? (See section [A.3.1].)

2   There is a radio programme of interest to the visually impaired. What is it called? When is it transmitted and what sort of topics does it cover? (See section [A.3.1.3].)

3   How would you find out what organisations are active in the area in which you live or work? (See section [A.3.1].)

4   How would you find out if there were a specialist group catering for the same particular hobby, etc., of interest to an individual patient? (See section [A.3.1].)

5   Large print and large symbol items might well be of interest to partially sighted people. What sort of things would you tell them about? (See section [A.3.2.1].)

6   How does a person obtain a talking book or a talking newspaper? (See section [A.3.2.2].)

APPENDIX 4
Lighting Terminology: CIBS Code 1984/ IES Code 1977

Luminous flux: The light emitted by a source or received by a surface.

Lumen (lm): Unit of luminous flux.

Luminous intensity: The quantity which describes the power of a source or illuminated surface to emit light in a given direction.

Candela (cd): Unit of luminous intensity; equal to 1 lumen/steradian.

Illumination: The process of lighting an object.

Illuminance: The luminous flux density at a surface, i.e. the luminous flux incident/unit area.

Lux: Unit of illuminance; equal to $1\,lm/m^2$, i.e. a surface 1 m away from a source of power 1 cd has an illuminance level of 1 lux.

Foot candle (ft cd or f.c.): unit of illuminance used in USA equal to $1\,lm/ft^2$.

Conversion: 1 lux = 0.093 ft cd; 1 ft cd = 10.76 lux

Luminance: Physical measure of intensity of light emitted in a given direction (usually towards the observer) by a unit area of a self luminous, transmitting or reflecting surface.

Apostilb or candela/m²: Unit of luminance.

Some examples to give a sense of scale (adapted from Jay, 1978):

Luminous flux: A single wax candle emits approximately 12 lumens in total. It is therefore equivalent to a 1 W filament bulb, since a 100 W filament bulb emits approximately 1200 lumens in total.

Luminous intensity: 100 W bulb gives 100 cd in all directions, compared to a 100 W reflector spotlight which has the same total light output, but concentrates the light in one direction giving 3000 cd in the centre of the beam.

APPENDIX 5
Suppliers of Optical and Electronic Visual Aids

Alpha Vision,
North's Estate,
Piddington,
High Wycombe,
Bucks HP12 3BE
Tel: 01494 883838

CCTV and electronic systems.

Associated Optical,
Unit 2, 64 High St,
Burnham,
Bucks SL1 7JT
Tel: 01628 605433

Eschenbach range of magnifiers and telescopes.

Claritas Ltd,
2 Earlswood St,
Greenwich,
London SE10 9ES
Tel: 0181 858 2411

Magnifiers and telescopes.

Combined Optical Industries Ltd,
200 Bath Rd,
Slough,
Berks SL1 4DW
Tel: 01753 75011

Magnifiers, telescopes and hyperocular lenses.

Concept Systems,
204–206 Queens Rd,
Beeston,
Nottingham NG9 8AL
Tel: 0115 925 5988

CCTV systems.

Dept of Health and Human Services,
National Eye Institute,
Building 31,
Bethesda,
Maryland, USA

Force Ten Company Ltd,
183 Boundary Rd,
Woking,
Surrey GU21 5BU
Tel: 01483 762711

Eezee writer and Eezee reader.

Globe Screen Printing,
875 Hollins St,
Baltimore, MD 21201, USA

Ferris Visual Acuity Charts.

Horizon
11 Lowman Units,
Tiverton Business Park,
Tiverton,
Devon EX16 6SR
Tel: 01884 254172

Magnifiers, telescopes and CCTV systems.

Keeler Ltd,
Clewer Hill Rd,
Windsor,
Berks SL4 4AA
Tel: 01753 857177

Telescopic units, magnifiers.

Lighthouse Optical Aids Division,
111 East 59th St,
New York, NY 10022,
USA

Edward Marcus Ltd,
14 Goswell Rd,
London EC1M 7AA
Tel: 0171 490 5915

Magnifiers and telescopes.

Norville Group,
Magdala Rd,
Gloucester GL1 4DG
Tel: 0145 252 8686

PLS lens tints.

Optima Low Vision Services,
Bluecoat School House,
Totnes,
Devon TQ9 5SP
Tel: 01803 864218

CCTV supply.

Professional Vision Services,
90 Walsworth Rd,
Hitchin,
Herts SG4 9SX
Tel: 01462 420751

CCTV supply.

Rodenstock UK (Lens Division),
Springhead Rd,
Northfleet,
Kent DA11 6HJ
Tel: 01474 325555

Lambda 660 block filter lens.

School of Optometry,
University of California,
Berkeley,
CA 94720, USA

School of Optometry,
University of Waterloo,
Waterloo,
Ontario N2L 3G1, Canada

Sensory System Ltd,
1 Watling Gate,
297–303 Edgeware Rd,
London NW9 6NB
Tel: 0181 205 3002

CCTV and electronic equipment.

Specialist Optical Source,
57 Dukes Wood Drive,
Gerrards Cross,
Bucks SL9 7LJ
Tel: 01753 888411

Magnifiers, including LHP and
Schweizer range.

Sussex Vision,
Unit 16,
Winston Business Centre,
Chartwell Rd,
Lancing,
West Sussex BN15 8TU
Tel: 01903 851951

Magnifiers, telescopic spectacle units.

Thousand and One Lamps Ltd,
4 Barmeston Rd,
London SE6 3BN
Tel: 0181 698 7238

Lamps, copyholders, illuminated stand
magnifiers.

Viking Optical Ltd,
Blyth Rd,
Halesworth,
Suffolk IP19 8EN
Tel: 01986 875315

Magnifiers and telescopes.

Visualeyes,
19 Turn Lea,
Midgley,
Halifax,
West Yorks HX2 6TT
Tel: 01422 884689

CCTV systems.

Zeiss (Oberkochen) Ltd,
PO Box 78,
Woodfield Rd,
Welwyn Garden City,
Herts AL7 1LV
Tel: 01707 331144

Own design spectacle mounted
telescopic units.

APPENDIX 6

Useful Addresses: Support and Advisory Organisations

The Albino Fellowship,
Mark Sanderson,
9 Burnley Rd,
Hampton,
Burnley B11 5QR
Tel: 01282 776145

Association of Blind Chartered
Physiotherapists,
Mrs M. Fairbrother,
22 Ermine Way,
Stamford, Lincs PE9 2XN

Association of Blind and Partially
Sighted Teachers and Students,
BM Box 6727,
London WC1N 3XX

British Blind Sport,
67 Albert St,
Rugby CV21 2SN
Tel: 01788 536142

All matters relating to sports and leisure
time activities for visually impaired.

British Computer Association of the
Blind,
c/o 5 Windle Ct,
Locking Stumps,
Warrington, Cheshire

British Diabetic Association,
10 Queen Anne St,
London W1M 0BD
Tel: 0171 323 1531

British Journal of Visual Impairment,
Editorial Office,
55 Eton Ave,
London NW3 3ET
Tel: 0171 722 9703

British Retinitis Pigmentosa Society,
PO Box 350,
Buckingham MK18 5EL
Tel: 01280 860363

Calibre,
Aylesbury,
Bucks HP22 5XQ
Tel: 01296 432339

Talking book service.

Chivers Press Publishers,
Windsor Bridge Rd,
Bath BA2 3AX
Tel: 01225 335336

Publishers of the Lythway, New Portway,
Atlantic and Windsor range of large print
books. Agents for G.K. Hall American
books. Also a range of adult and
children's audio books.

Clio Press Ltd,
55 St Thomas Street,
Oxford OX1 1JG
Tel: 01865 250333

Publishers of ISIS, Landmark,
Masterworks, Windrush and
Cornerstone large print books and audio
books.

Disabled Living Foundation,
380–384 Harrow Rd,
London W9 2HU
Tel: 0171 289 6111

Major advice and information centre
with displays of RNIB and commercial
aids, LVAs and the *In Touch* kitchen.

Gardening for the Blind: Horticultural
Therapy,
Goulds Grounds,
Vallis Way,
Frome,
Somerset BA11 3DW
Tel: 01373 467072

International Glaucoma Association,
c/o Mrs Wright,
Kings College Hospital,
Denmark Hill,
London SE5 9RS
Tel: 0171 737 3265

Jewish Care,
221 Golders Green Rd,
London NW11 9DN
Tel: 0181 458 3282

Library Association,
7 Ridgemount St,
London WC1E 7AE
Tel: 0171 636 7543

Information leaflets.

LOOK (National Federation of Families
with Visually Impaired Children),
c/o Queen Alexandra College,
Court Oak Rd,
Birmingham B17 9TG
Tel: 0121 428 5038

Macular Disease Society,
PO Box 247,
Haywards Heath,
West Sussex RH17 5FF
Tel: 01990 143573

Magna Print Books,
Magna House,
Long Preston,
Skipton,
North Yorks BD23 4ND
Tel: 01729 840225

National Deaf-Blind League,
18 Rainbow Ct,
Paston Ridings,
Peterborough PE4 6UP
Tel: 01733 73511

National Library for the Blind,
Cromwell Rd,
Bredbury,
Stockport SK6 2SG
Tel: 0161 494 0217

National Federation of the Blind,
Unity House,
Smythe St,
Westgate,
Wakefield, West Yorks WF1 1ER

Northern Ireland Blind Centre,
70 North Rd,
Belfast BT5 5NJ
Tel: 01232 654366

Partially Sighted Society,
PO Box 322,
Doncaster DN1 2XA
Tel: 01302 323132

Mail order, membership, publications, printing, enlarging.

PSS Greater London Office (general enquiries),
62 Salisbury Rd,
London NW6 6RH
Tel: 0171 372 1551

PSS Sight Centres – low vision advice, training and information.

Exeter: Dean Clarke House,
Southernhay East,
Exeter EX1 1PE
Tel: 01392 210656

Salisbury: District Hospital,
Salisbury SP2 8BJ
Tel: 01722 336262

Royal National Institute for the Blind (RNIB),
Head office – general enquiries,
224 Gt Portland St,
London W1A 6AA
Tel: 0171 388 1266

RNIB Talking Book Service,
Mount Pleasant,
Wembley,
Middlesex HA0 1RR
Tel: 0181 903 6666

St Dunstan's,
PO Box 4XB,
12–14 Harcourt St,
London W1A 4XB
Tel: 0171 723 5021

Scottish National Federation for the Welfare of the Blind,
PO Box 500,
Gillespie Crescent,
Edinburgh EH10 4HZ
Tel: 0131 229 1456

SENSE (National Association for Deaf/ Blind and Rubella Handicapped),
11–13 Clifton Terrace,
London N4 3SR
Tel: 0171 272 7774

Talking Newspaper Association of the United Kingdom,
National Recording Centre,
Heathfield,
East Sussex TN21 8DB
Tel: 01435 866102

Tape Recording Service for the Blind,
24 Catherine St,
Dumfries DG1 1HZ
Tel: 01387 53927

Torch Trust for the Blind,
Torch House,
Hallaton,
Market Harborough,
Leics LE16 8UJ
Tel: 01858 555301

Ulverscroft Large Print Books Ltd,
The Green,
Bradgate Rd,
Anstey,
Leics LE7 7FU
Tel: 01533 364325

Wales Council for the Blind,
Shand House,
20 Newport Rd,
Cardiff CF2 1YB
Tel: 01222 473954

Warwickshire Association for the Blind,
George Marshall Centre,
Puckerings Lane,
Warwick CV2 4UH
Tel: 01926 494129

References

Abadi, R.V. (1979) 'Visual performance with contact lenses and congenital idiopathic nystagmus'. *Br. J. Physiol. Opt.*, **33**, 32–7.

Abadi, R.V. and Sandikcioglu, M. (1975) 'Visual resolution in congenital pendular nystagmus'. *Amer. J. Optom. Physiol. Opt.*, **52**, 573–81.

Adrian, W., Everson, R.W. and Schmidt, I. (1977) 'Protection against photic damage in retinitis pigmentosa'. In *RP: clinic implications of current research*, (Ed. by Landers, M.B., Wolbarsht, M.L., Dowling, J.E. and Laties, A.M.). Plenum Press, New York.

Arden, G.B. & Jacobson, J. (1978) 'A simple grating test for contrast sensitivity'. *Invest. Ophthalmol. Vis. Sci.*, 23–32.

Armstrong, J.R., Daily, R.K., Dobson, H.L. and Girard, L.J. (1960) 'The incidence of glaucoma in diabetes mellitus'. *Amer. J. Ophthal.*, **50**, 55.

Atkinson, J. and Braddick, O. (1984) 'Screening for refractive errors in 6–9 month old infants by photorefraction'. *Brit. J. Ophthal.*, **68**, 105–12.

Atkinson, J., Braddick, O. and Pimm-Smith, E. (1982) 'Preferential looking monocular and binocular acuity test in infants'. *Brit. J. Ophthal.*, **66**, 264–8.

Atkinson, J., Braddick, O., Pimm-Smith, E., Ayling, L. and Sawyer, R. (1981) 'Does the Catford Drum give an accurate assessment of acuity?'. *Brit. J. Ophthal.*, **65**, 652–6.

Backman, O. and Inde, K. (1979) *Low vision training*. Liber Harmods, Malmo, Sweden.

Bailey, I.L. (1978) 'Visual field measurement in low Vision'. *Optometric Monthly*, **69**, 697–701.

Bailey, I.L. (1978) 'Field expander'. *Optometric Monthly*, **69**, 813–16.

Bailey, I.L. (1978) 'Prismatic treatment for field defects'. *Optometric Monthly*, **69**, 1073–1078.

Bailey, I.L. (1980) 'Magnification for near vision'. *Optometric Monthly*, **71**, 119–22.

Bailey, I.L. (1980) 'Combining accommodation with spectacle additions'. *Optometric Monthly*, **71**, 397–9.

Bailey, I.L. (1980) 'Combining hand magnifiers and spectacle additions'. *Optometric Monthly*, **71**, 458–61.

Bailey, I.L. (1981) 'Verifying near vision magnifiers'. Part 1 *Optometric Monthly*, **72** (1), 42–3; Part 2 *Optometric Monthly*, **72** (2), 34–8.

Bailey, I.L. (1981) 'Locating the image in stand magnifiers'. *Optometric Monthly*, **72** (6), 22–4.

Bailey, I.L. (1981) 'The use of fixed focus stand magnifiers'. *Optometric Monthly*, **72** (8), 37–9.

Bailey, I.L. (1982) 'Mirrors for visual field defects'. *Optometric Monthly*, **73**, 202–206.

Bailey, I.L. and Lovie, J.E. (1976) 'New design principles for visual acuity letter charts'. *Amer. J. Optom. Physiol. Opt.*, **53**, 740–45.

Bailey, I.L. and Lovie, J.E. (1980) 'Design and use of a new near vision chart'. *Amer. J. Optom. Physiol. Opt.*, **57**, 378–87.

Bennett, A.G. (1975) 'Igard hyperoculars, their design and development'. *Ophth. Optician*, **15**, 1151–4.

Bennett, A.G. (1977) 'Review of ophthalmic standards'. Part II. Hand and stand magnifiers. *Manuf. Opt. Int.*, **30**, 67–73.

Bennett, A.G. (1982) 'Spectacle magnification and loupe magnification'. *Optician*, **183**, (4740), 16–18, 36.

Bennett, A.G. and Rabbetts, R.B. (1984) in *Clinical Visual Optics*. Butterworths, London.

Bier, N. (1970) *Correction of subnormal vision*, 2nd edn., p. 102. Butterworths, London.

Bier, N. and Lowther, G.E. (1977) in *Contact Lens Correction*, p. 483–7. Butterworths, London.

Blakemore, C. and Campbell, F.W. (1969) on 'The existence of neurons in the human visual system selectively sensitive to the orientation and size of retinal images'. *J. Physiol.*, **203**, 237–60.

Boyce, P.R. (1978) 'Relationship between performance of visual tasks and lighting conditions' Light for Low Vision Symposium, University College, London.

Campbell, F.W. and Maffei, L. (1974) 'Contrast and spatial frequency'. *Sci. Am.*, **231**, 106–14.

CIBS Code for Interior Lighting (1984) 5th edn. Chartered Institution of Building Services Engineers – Lighting Division, London.

Collins, J. (1987) 'Coping with the rising incidence of partial sight'. *Optometry Today*, **27**, 772–9.

Cuifreda, K.J. (1977) 'A new field expander *Optom. Weekly*, **68**, 29–30.

Dallos, J. (1936) 'Contact glasses: the "Invisible" spectacles'. *Arch. Ophthal.*, 15 April. p. 617.

Ditmars, D.L. and Keener, R.J. (1976) 'A contact lens for the treatment of colour vision defects'. *Military Med.*, **141**, 319–22.

Dowie, A.T. (1988) *Management and practice of low visual acuity*. Association of British Dispensing Opticians, London.

Drasdo, N. and Murray, I.J. (1978) 'Pilot study of the use of visual field expanders'. *Br. J. Physiol. Opt.*, **32**, 22–9.

Duke Elder, S. (1964) in 'System of Ophthalmology'. **III**, Part 2, *Congenital Deformities*. Henry Kimpton, London.

Duke Elder, S. (1967) In 'System of Ophthalmology'. **X**, *Diseases of the Retina*. Henry Kimpton, London.

Edwards, K.H. (1988) in *Optometry. Part 3* (Ed. by Edwards, K.H. and Llewellyn, R.D.). Butterworths, London.

Eger, M.J. (1974) 'The X-CHROM Lens Case Reports'. *J. Amer. Optom. Assoc.*, **45**, 81–7.

Elliot, D. (1988) 'Is 6/6 good enough?' *Optician*, **196**, (5164), 18–20.

Elliott, R. (1985) 'A new linear picture vision test'. *Brit. Orthopt. J.*, **42**, 54–7.

Everson, R.W. and Schmidt, I. (1976) 'Protective spectacles for retinitis pigmentosa patients'. *J. Amer. Optom. Assoc.*, **47**, 738–44.

Faye, E.E. (1984) Clinical Low Vision, 2nd edn. Little, Brown and Company, Boston.

Faye, E.E. (1986) in *Low Vision: Principles and Applications* (Ed. by George Woo). Springer-Verlag, New York.

Ferris, F.L., Kassoff, A., Bresnick, G.H. and Bailey, I. (1982) 'New visual acuity charts for clinical research'. *Amer. J. Ophthal.*, **94**, 91–6.

Fletcher, R. (1979) 'Evaluation of a CCTV device for partial sight'. *Br. J. Physiol. Opt.*, **33**, 11–18.

Fletcher, R. and Voke, J. (1985) *Defective Colour Vision*. Adam Hilger, Bristol & Boston.

Fonda, G. (1962) 'Characteristics and Low Vision correction in albinism'. *Arch. Ophthal.*, **68**, 754–60.

Fonda, G. (1978) 'Binocular reading additions for low vision'. *Arch. Ophthal.*, **83**, 294–9.

Fonda, G. (1981) in *Management of Low Vision*. Thieme-Stratton Inc, N.Y.

Foulds, W. (1980) 'Factors influencing visual recovery in retinal detachment surgery'. *Trans. Ophthal. Soc.*, UK 100, 72–7.

Gartner, S. and Henkind, P. (1981) 'Ageing and degeneration of the human macula. 1. Outer nuclear layer and photoreceptors'. *Brit. J. Ophthal.*, **65**, 23–8.

Gill, J.M. (1983) 'Survey of Reading Stands'. *Ophth. Optician.*, **23**, 38–40.

Gill, J. and Silver, J.H. (1982) 'Illumination from domestic lamps'. *Ophth. Optician.*, **22**, 282.

Ginsburg, A.P. (1984) 'A New Contrast Sensitivity Vision Test Chart'. *Amer. J. Optom. Physiol. Opt.*, **61**, 403–407.

Goodrich, G.L. and Quillman, R.D. (1977) 'Training Eccentric Viewing'. *J. Vis. Impair. Blind.*, **71**, 377–81.

Graham, N. (1981) 'Psychophysics of Spatial Frequency Channels'. In *Perceptual Organisation* 2nd edn. (Ed. by Kubovy and Pomerantz) 1–25. Embalm, New Jersey.

Grenensky, S.M. (1969) 'Some comments on a closed circuit TV system for the visually handicapped' *Amer. J. Optom.*, **46**, 519–24.

Grenensky, S.M., Peterson, H.E., Moshin, H.L., Clewett, R.W. and Yoshimura, R.I. (1972) 'Advances in closed circuit TV systems for the partially sighted'. Rand. Santa-Monica R-1040. HEW/RCA.

Hess, R.F. (1984) 'The assessment of contrast threshold functions for anomalous vision'. *Br. Orthopt. J.*, **41**, 1–14.

Hess, R.F. (1986) in *Low Vision: Principles and Applications* (Ed. by George Woo). Springer-Verlag, New York.

Hoyt, C.S., Jastrzgbski, G.B. and Marg, E. (1983) 'Delayed visual maturation in infancy'. *Brit. J. Ophthal.*, **67**, 127–30.

IES Code for Interior Lighting (1977), Illuminating Engineering Society (London).

Jackson, J. and Silver, J. (1983) 'Visual Disability. Part 4: Spectacle and head-borne magnifiers'. *Ophth. Optician*, **23**, 214–23.

Jay, Peter (1978) '*Fundamentals*': paper presented at the 'Light for Low Vision' Symposium, University College, London.

Julian, W.G. (1984) 'Variation in near visual acuity with illuminance for a group of 27 partially sighted people'. *Lighting Res. and Technology*, **16**, (i) 34–41.

Kay, H. (1983) 'A new method of assessing VA with pictures'. *Brit. J. Ophthal.*, **67**, 131–3.

Keeler, C.H. (1956) *Trans. Ophth. Soc. UK*, **76**, 605.

Keeler, C.H. (1968) *Helping the Partially Sighted – Manual* 5th edn. Keeler, London.

Klein, D., Franceschetti, A., Hussles, I., Race, R:R. and Sanger, R. (1967) 'X-linked Retinitis Pigmentosa Linkage Studies with the Xg Blood Groups'. *The Lancet*, **1**, 974.

Krill, A.E. and Deutman, A.F. (1972) 'The various categories of juvenile macular disease'. *Trans. Amer. Ophthal. Soc.*, **70**, 220.

La Bissoniere, P.E. (1974) 'The X-CHROM Lens' *Int. Contact Lens Clinic*, 1/4, 48–55.

Law, F.W. (1952) 'Reading Types'. *Brit. J. Ophthal.*, **36**, 689.

Lebensohn, J.E. (1949) 'Practical problems relating to presbyopia'. *Amer. J. Ophthal.*, **32**, 22.

Levitt, J. (1978) 'Lighting for the elderly – an optician's view': paper presented at the 'Light for Low Vision' Symposium, University College, London.

Mandell, R.B. (1965) *Contact Lens Practice, basic and advanced*. Thomas, Springfield.

Mann, I. (1957) Developmental Abnormalities of the Eye 2nd edn. Lippincott, Philadelphia.

Marshall, J. (1977) 'The Retinal receptors and the pigment epithelium'. In *Scientific Foundations of Ophthalmology* (Ed. by Perkins, E.S. and Hill, D.W.) Heineman, London.

Marshall, J. (1985) 'Radiation and Ageing Eye'. *Ophthal. Physiol. Opt.*, **5**, 241–63.

McKusick, V. (1968) 'Mendelian inheritance in man'. In *Catologs of Autosomal Dominant, Autosomal Recessive and X-linked phenotypes*, 2nd Edn. Johns Hopkins Press, Baltimore.

Michaelson, I.C. (1980) Disorders at the Macula. In *Textbook of the Fundus of the Eye* 3rd edn. Churchill Livingstone, London.

NAS – NRC Committee of Vision (1980) 'Recommended standard procedures for the clinical measurement and specification of visual acuity'. *Adv. Ophthal.*, **41**, 103.

Nissenhorn, I., Yassur, Y., Maskowski, D., Sherf, I. and Bensira, I. (1983) 'Myopia in premature babies with and without retinopathy of prematurity'. *Brit. J. Ophthal.*, **67**, 170–73.

Noell, W.K., Walker, V.S., Kang, B.S. and Berman, S. (1966) 'Damage by light in rats'. *Invest. Ophthal. Vis. Sci.*, **5**, 450–73.

Pelli, D.G., Robson, J.G. & Wilkins, A.J. (1988) 'The design of a new chart for measuring contrast sensitivity'. *Clin. Vis. Sci*, **2**, 187–99.

Potts, A.M., Volk, D. and West, S.S. (1959) 'A television reader as a subnormal vision aid' *Amer. J. Ophthal.*, **47**, 580–81.

Reeves, B. (1991) 'The Pelli–Robson low contrast letter chart'. *Optician*, **201** (59292) 18–27.

Reeves, B.C. and Hill, A.R. (1987) 'Practical problems in measuring contrast sensitivity'. Part I. *Optician*, **193**, (5085), 29–34; Part II. *Optician*, **193**, (5086), 30–34.

Regan, D. and Neima, D. (1983) 'Low contrast letter charts as tests of visual function'. *Ophthalmology*, **90**, 1192–1200.

Ruben, M. (1967) 'Albinism and Contact Lenses' *Contact Lens Journal*, **1**, 5–8.

Rumney, N.J. (1989) 'An Improved Range of Low Vision Aids'. Part I, *Optician*, **198**, (5221) 28–31; Part II: *Optician*, **198**, (5227) 11–13.

Sarks, S.H. (1976) 'Ageing and degeneration in the macular region: A Clinico-pathological study'. *Brit. J. Ophthal.*, **60**, 324–41.

Schmidt, I. (1976) 'Visual aids for correction of red–green colour deficiencies'. *Can. J. Optom.*, **38**, 38–47. (Reprinted *Optician*, 1977, 173, 7–35).

Shaw, A. (1969) 'Print for Partial Sight': a report to the Library Association Sub-committee on Books for Readers with Defective Sight. Library Association, London.

Siegel, I.M. (1981) 'The X-CHROM lens: On seeing red'. *Surv. Ophthal.*, **25**, 312–23.

Silver, J.H. (1976) 'Low vision aids in the management of visual handicap'. *Br. J. Physiol. Opt.*, **31**, 47.

Silver, J.H. (1979) 'Tinted lenses in retinitis pigmentosa'. *Optician*, **178**, (4618), 11–14.

Silver, J.H. (1985) Visual Disability. In *Optometry* (Ed. by Edwards, K. and Llewellyn, R.), Butterworth, London.

Silver, J. and Fass, V.H. (1977) 'CC TV as a low vision aid development and application'. *Ophthal. Optician*, **15**, 596–602.

Silver, J.H. and Gill, J.M. (1979) 'CC TV in use as an aid to employment'. *Ophthal. Optician*, **19**, 494–500.

Silver, J.H., Gould, E.S., Irvine, D. and Cullinan, T.R. (1978) 'Visual Acuity at home and in eye clinics'. *Trans. Ophthal. Soc.*, (UK) **98**, 262. Reprinted. *Ophthal. Optician* (1980) **20**, 106–111.

Silver, J.H. and Lyness, A.L. (1985) 'Do retinitis pigmentosa patients prefer red photochromic lenses?' *Ophthal. Physiol. Opt.*, **5**, 87–9.

Silver, J.H. and Woodward, E.G. (1978) 'Driving with a visual disability'. *Ophthal. Optician*, **18**, 794–5.

Sloan, L.L. (1959) 'New test chart for the measurement of visual acuity at far and near distances'. *Amer. J. Ophthal.*, **48**, 807.

Sloan, L.L. and Brown, D.J. (1963) 'Reading cards for the selection of optical aids for the partially sighted'. *Amer. J. Ophthal.*, **55**, 1187.

Sloan, L.L. and Habel, A. (1956) 'Reading Aids for the partially blind'. *Amer. J. Ophthal.*, **42**, 863.

Sloan, L., Habel, A. and Feiock, K. (1973) 'High illumination as an auxiliary reading aid in diseases of the macula'. *Amer. J. Ophthal.*, **76**, 745.

Sorsby, A. (1966) *The incidence and causes of blindness in England and Wales. 1948−62.* HMSO, London.

Sorsby, A. (1979) *Blindness and partial sight in England 1969/70.* DHSS reports on Public Health and Medical Subjects No 129. DHSS, London.

Stone, J. and Breakspear, H. (1977) 'Two interesting cases of low visual acuity seen at the London Refraction Hospital'. *Contact Lens Journal*, **6**, 3−6.

Strong, G. and Woo, G. (1985) 'A distance visual acuity chart incorporating some new design features'. *Arch. Ophthal.*, **103**, 44−6.

Tarizzo, M.L. (1972) 'The role of the World Health Organisation in the prevention of blindness'. *Proceedings of Jerusalem Seminar on the Prevention of Blindness.* Academic Press, New York.

Taylor, S.P. (1979) 'The use of tinted lenses as aids in the treatment of pigmentary retinal degeneration − a review'. *Br. J. Physiol. Opt.*, **33**, 38−43.

Taylor, S.P. (1984) 'The X-CHROM lens − patients see red!' *Optician*, 187 (4944) 24−34.

The *In Touch* Handbook 6th edn. (1989) Broadcasting Support Services, PO Box 7, London, W3 6XJ.

Trevor Roper, P.D. (1952) 'Marriage of two complete albinos with normally pigmented offspring'. *Brit. J. Ophthal.*, **36**, 107.

Tunnacliffe, A. (1989) 'A new clinical contrast sensitivity test'. *Optician*, **197**, (5185), 13−18.

Waardenburg, P.J., Franceschetti, A. and Klein, D. (1961) *Genetics and Ophthalmology.* Blackwell Scientific Publication Oxford.

Weale, R.A. (1963) *The Ageing Eye.* Lewis, London.

Weiss, N.J. (1972) 'An application of cemented prisms with severe field loss'. *Amer. J. Optom.*, **49**, 261−4.

Weston, H.C. (1961) Trans IES (London) 26, 1.

Wilkins, A. (1986) 'Contrast sensitivity and its measurements'. *Optician*, 192, (5054), 13−14.

Zeltzer, H.I. (1971) 'The X-CHROM lens'. *J. Am. Optom. Ass.*, **42**, 933−7.

Index